I'd Rather Have Cancer

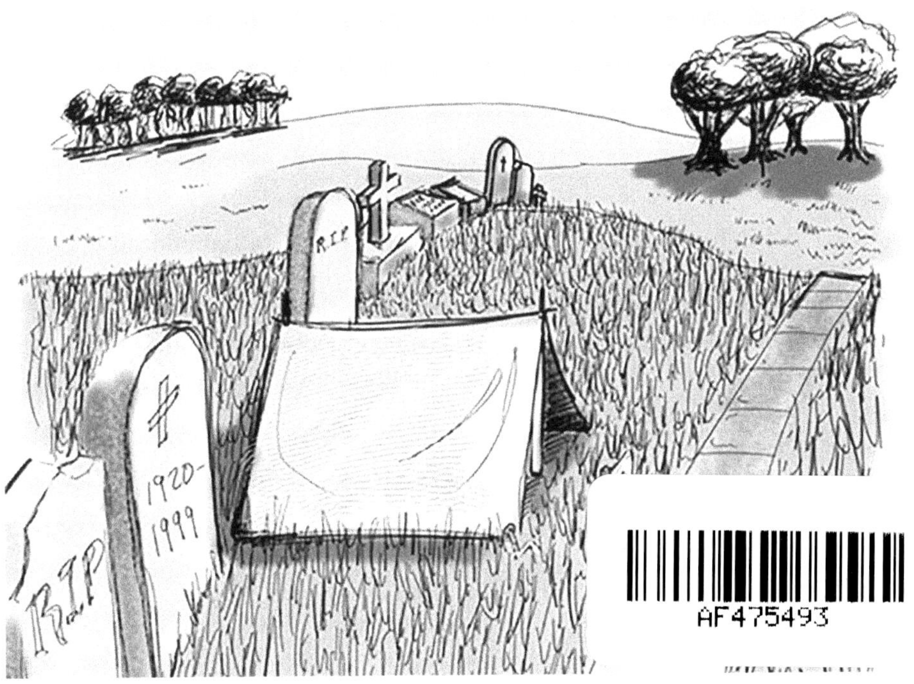

By Stephen Butterman
Illustrated by Adam Frizzell

Bellissima Publishing, LLC
Jamul, California
www.bellissimapublishing.com

IBSN 978-1-61477-248-4
First Edition

"The fear of death follows from the fear of life. A man who lives fully is prepared to die at any time."

MARK TWAIN

To Penny Weigand--publisher, editor, songstress, and friend.

CHAPTER ONE

OUT OF THE FRYING PAN AND INTO THE SLOW BURNER

We are all in the gutter, but some of us are looking at the stars.
~ Oscar Wilde

The last time that I had sat in this drab blue examination room, it had transformed into a scene of triumph. This had been all the sweeter because on all of my other previous visits here, I had experienced disappointment and anxiety—first, because my salivary gland cancer had spread, then, time and again, because the cancer had not gone away, meaning more trips to the "chemo suite" down the hall, more hair-loss, exhaustion, nausea, constipation.

At last, two months ago my oncologist had happily informed me that my most recent CT-scan revealed no cancer. We defeated the killer, meaning no more chemo, no more hair-loss, exhaustion, nausea, constipation.

So why had I returned to this room two months later? Earlier in the day I had underwent a standard echocardiogram of my heart "just to be safe" as Doc had worded it, and he wanted to see me afterward to discuss the presumably routine results.

You see, alongside all of the irritating *temporary* side effects of chemo—weight-loss and hair-loss, for example—a longer-term effect of my particular chemo-cocktail was that it weakens heart muscles. Having been blessed with a naturally strong heart, I had not worried much about that. I figured it could afford some weakening and yet remain relatively strong. People in my genetic line generally do not fall to heart attacks.

I considered *all* of chemo's side-effects to be things of the past. My hair was growing back, and *without* any grey; my belly was also making a comeback, and I now affectionately patted it.

Finally, in came Doc, a tall meaty man with oily skin and with a lick of dark hair swirled about his broad forehead. His smile of greeting seemed strained, nothing like the warm and triumphant smile of my last visit. Instead of sitting down as usual, he began pacing as he began talking.

"I will be referring you to one of our top cardiologists. However, I *can* tell you now that your echocardiogram reveals that the ejection fraction on your right ventricle is below 30, whereas normal is 50," he said stoically.

"Sounds like something a car mechanic could fix," I quipped, smiling. "What does it mean?"

Doc did not smile back.

He swiped his hand across his lick of unruly hair, paced a couple of steps and, facing me, said, "Your cardiologist will explain this in detail, and will treat it accordingly, but that E.F. means that you have severe congestive heart failure."

He sank into a chair.

"Jeez, Doc. Heart *failure*? That sounds *serious*!"

"You had mentioned 'mild' shortness of breath?" he asked, wrinkling his lick-covered brow.

"Yea, just the past couple months. I should *never* have smoked!"

"Well, that breathing trouble is likely caused by fluid in your lungs. Your right ventricle is the one that pumps out blood, but yours is only pumping out 50-60 percent of what it should each heartbeat; that means you'll have a fluid back-up in your lungs, hence a shortness of breath, especially lying down."

"Lying *down*?" I squeaked, suddenly panicked by a vision of me in a coffin that I could ill afford on my income. "Doc, am I *dying?* After whipping cancer?"

He finally smiled more like he had on my last visit.

"Oh no! They have drugs now—your cardiologist will take care of you—that can greatly extend the lives of people with your problem. And, those meds have *nothing* like the side-effects of chemo drugs."

"You mean they won't cause cancer?"

"Ha-ha, no!" He patted my arm reassuringly. "I suppose you could live for *decades.*"

(Just this morning I had been thinking of living for *centuries*, me the all-powerful cancer-vanquisher!)

"Of course, you'll want to establish some lifestyle changes. *Moderation*—in eating, in drinking, in physical activity—should be your motto from now on: moderation in all things!"

Starting to feel a tad peevish, I slouched further into my chair.

"It seems maybe we should have used a little more moderation with the chemo, eh, Doc?"

He patted my slouched shoulder and headed toward the door.

"Well, at least we and that chemo whipped cancer, right? It also helped that you always stayed so *positive*. Why not call this new issue 'congestive heart *challenge*'?"

I could not smile at the moment, but I said, and meant it, "Good to see you, Doc."

Later at home I would feel some rage, but I quickly reminded myself to be *moderate* about it and the alcohol that would accompany it. I had always enjoyed traveling the road of excess, had always thought it the only road for a writer. How could one live life to the fullest in a moderate way? My newly compromised life and style seemed likely to slip into a quicksand pit of contradictions.

Popping open another beer, I thought back to the days of battling cancer, with moderation in *no* things. Ah, those were the days …

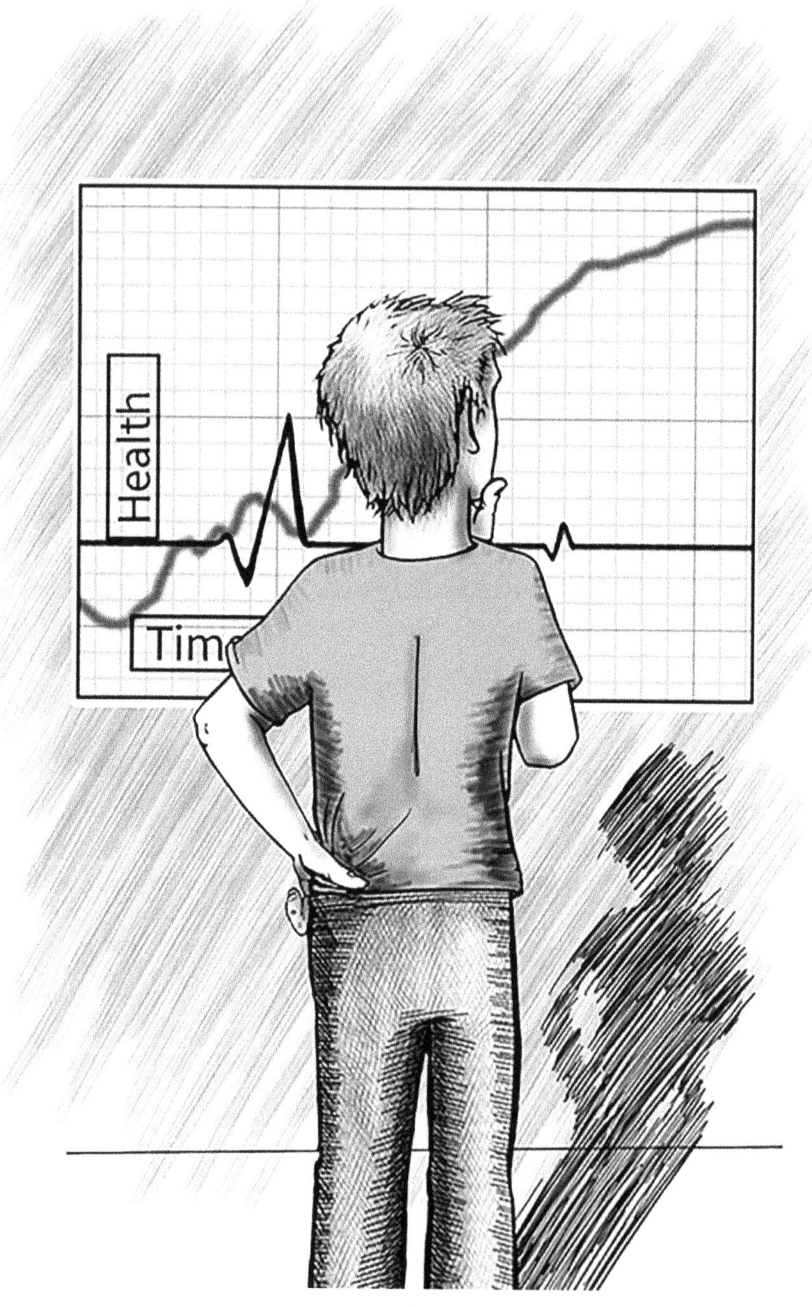
Health

CHAPTER TWO

I'D RATHER HAVE CANCER

Bygone troubles are good to tell.
~ Yiddish proverb

In short, I'd rather have cancer. That may seem a strange choice, not that I *chose* either, but I have had both cancer and heart failure—unless you have had both, you will have to take my word for it. Right off, the cancer experience ~~is~~ was way more fun.

For example, I had a blast writing my book (*That's So Funny, My Hair Fell Out!*) about cancer, enjoying it so much that this book will also be kind of about cancer. It had been stress-free writing about kicking cancer's ass while doing just that because cancer patients—writers among them—can make merry with the topic. While heart issues dampen passions, cancer rouses passions such as love and hate. Cancer is something that we *love* to hate and something that we love poking fun at. right? You can see the truth of that in the titles of *funny books about cancer*—a search-phrase that results in over 500 titles at amazon.com. I am not saying, and I will never say, that any of those books are as good or as funny or as meaningful as my funny book about cancer—well, *maybe* as meaningful; nevertheless, consider the comic outlooks behind these titles of books by cancer patients:

- *Cancer Schmancer*
- *Where Would You Like Your Nipple?*
- *There's a Mass in My Ass*
- *When Good Boobs Turn Bad: A Mammoir*
- *Not Now, I'm having a No-Hair Day*

It is understandable that cancer activates the "one book in me" concept for many cancer patients, but why does it also make them fledgling comedians? Is this laughing instead of crying? Is this like shouting at the devil but with laughs supplanting shouts? I do not know, but I sure do approve!

By comparison, an amazon.com search for *funny books about heart disease* results in less than 50 titles, some of which are apparently not even about heart disease, and many of which do not even *sound* funny. I do, however, like the titles, *I Took a Lickin' and Kept on Tickin'* and *How to Have a Heart Attack in 8 Easy Steps.* I am sure that they would bring a smile or a chuckle. Then again, some of those funny cancer books would bring chortles, guffaws, and belly laughs. It seems that deadly cancer is a livelier subject. That is one *big* reason why I'd rather have cancer *and* say so in the title of this book.

Such books convince us of what we would not guess—that the experience of battling cancer can be fun. Cancer related gifts, especially tee-shirts, project the same point while also portraying cancer patients as tough customers.

Tee-shirts are just one category, albeit the largest one, of cancer-related products: flags, banners, candles, bracelets, necklaces, dog-tags, doo-rags, coffee mugs, teddy bears, night lights, throw pillows, and etcetera. Why so many cancer-theme products? For one thing, people like to buy gifts for cancer patients—another reason to rather have cancer! Also, the most popular of these products have pink-tinted breast-cancer themes; women do love to shop, after all, and men do love *anything* pertaining to breasts. Carcinogenic entrepreneurs are slyly making millions off of these basic facts.

Okay, back to cancer-theme tee-shirts and how they, in a good-humored way, make cancer patients look *tough.* Consider these tee-shirt phrases:

- **CANCER SUCKS**
- **F*CK CANCER** (a mild version of this is **F**K CANCER**, a milder version **F*** CANCER**, or, mildest of all, **** **CANCER**)

- **CHEMO NINJA CANCER ASSASSIN**
- **CANCER MESSED WITH THE WRONG GIRL**
- **DO NOT DISTURB: BUSY KICKING CANCER'S ASS**

These shirts do not invite hugs. They kind of say, *stay out of my way—I'm in a fighting mood!* Fights are undeniably interesting if not downright exciting.

Compare that feisty attitude to the bland tone of these comparatively boring heart-issue tees:

- **Still Ticking**
- **See, It Works**
- **The Beat Goes On**
- **Congestive Heart Failure Stinks**

Yawn! By comparing these tee-shirts, we can savvy that cancer patients are bad asses easily imagined in combat gear with weapons and that heart patients must wear footsies and use 'exercycles.' How do you fight a heart issue? Fighting is *stressful*, and heart issues mean you *must* avoid stress.

My heart issue "stinks" while cancer "sucks." Those cancer patients do *not* mince words! Saying "cancer sucks" is now socially acceptable. As a mantra, it is currently as popular as were the post-

9/11 "USA!" chants, or the "Go Tribe!" chants around Cleveland during baseball season, or the "Go Buckeyes!" chants throughout Ohio year-round. You can even overhear "Cancer sucks!" in rest homes and daycare centers. You would not normally wear a shirt saying that *anything* "sucks" to church, but I have spied **CANCER SUCKS** tee-shirts beneath sweaters and jackets on my infrequent church visits. One time, I even *thought* I heard, during a hypnotic prayer-response session, the preacher murmuring, "Cancer sucks" and the spellbound congregation feverishly responding "Amen" without missing a beat. Maybe it was just my imagination, maybe not . . .

Anyway, although it is relatively mild, I do like my **Still Ticking** tee. However, I need to exercise caution wearing it out in the summer when I am tan, especially since my chemo-caused baldness made me a wearer of do-rags, making me, technically, a rag-head—I could look somewhat like an Arab. I have feared that some auxiliary deputy-dog who thinks he or she is part of Homeland Security will see me looking Arabic and wearing a **Still Ticking** shirt, deducing that it signals a bomb ticking away somewhere near, conking me repeatedly with a club, perhaps tasering me for good measure, and promptly shipping my butt off to Guantanamo.

In a cell I would tick down, forlorn and forgotten—unless the prison doctors would have re-diagnosed me with cancer. All I would have to do in that case would have been to someway get on Facebook from Guantanamo.

Soon after that, the president, himself or herself, would personally pardon me just to find *relief* from a tidal wave of indignant protests sent by *zillions* of Facebookers who had befriended me *merely* because I had cancer and said so on Facebook.

You see, no matter how cool and popular I might have been in the past, I could never have even approximated the supersonic coolness and popularity that goes with the status of cancer patient, aka Cancer Warrior. I had had about 100 Facebook "friends" (mostly extended family) prior to actually getting cancer. Once I announced it on FB, the friend requests poured in—before my second chemo treatment, I had accumulated 671 Facebook friends.

And they hit the *like* button for every one of my posts. For instance, I once posted, "Puked on chemo this morning, but half-alive and recovering now;" and *this* earned 519 likes! On the other hand, far more recently, I posted about how I had been diagnosed with chemo-caused heart failure, but would live with it; and *this* gained only *four* likes, those from my four sisters! Suddenly, I see that I now have only 414 friends, oops, make that 405—404, 401, 393—and I cannot help to feel like a Facebook leper! *Goodbye, fair-cancer friends!*

So, those *were* the days! Smile, and the world smiles with you. Smile as a **CHEMO NINJA CANCER ASSASSIN,** and the world pats your back, buys you beers, offers you rides, and perhaps throws you a party.

I have done some *BIG* things in my life—cross-country bicycle tours, writing books, and so forth—but I never attained fame for performing those actions like for getting cancer. This often-fatal affliction can make you a cultural star in general, and a *Super Star* at benefit bashes thrown for you, big bashes where friends, family, and total strangers get smashed, whoop it up, and toss money around—all in honor of *you*, the fortunate one who came down with cancer which, as we all know, s*cks.

Missing all of that, feeling lately like not just my heart has been missing a beat, I attempted to rekindle the floundering flame of that old glory by attending a "Relay for Life" walkathon event where I would not be The Star, but a star among many stars. All about me at a local school's athletic complex, people were smiling—about cancer! Or at least about the communal spirit aligned against it, which is indeed awesome. Good luck getting such a spirited gathering in defense against congestive heart failure!

It was a smooth operation, with the slick corporate logo of the American Cancer Society everywhere evident, including on the trinkets and tee-shirts given to participants. As an official cancer "survivor," I received one of the purple tees with *FINISH THE FIGHT* on its front and *I AM HOPE* on its back—yea, hope that someday we might conquer cancer with something other than chemicals that savage our hearts and bodies.

Early in the crisp, mid-spring evening, we of the purple shirts walked a "survivor lap" around the all-weather track. The cancer-related comradery was *everywhere* apparent, as people lining the inside of the track clapped and cheered all of the way around, as if celebrating our victories over cancer. I walked with my niece Reggie, a true breast-cancer survivor and my hero during my own fight against cancer; yet, instead of what I *had* felt like just a few weeks previous—like a cancer-vanquishing champ—I now felt like an imposter the entire way. So, I let Reggie's fantastic smile suffice for both of us. I did not feel like smiling, did not feel victorious.

Shortly after the lap, I changed back into my **Still Ticking** shirt and Reggie changed back into her **CANCER SUCKS** shirt, which she wore with a smile.

Walking that lap had honestly winded me. I had wanted to get back into shape, but I had forgotten to ask my cardiologist about exercise guidelines on my first visit with him. I had more pressing questions like "*how long have I got*?"

Near the bustling concession stand where volunteers were grilling aromatic burgers and bratwursts, I encountered an old high school buddy, Jerry, wearing a tee-shirt just like Reggie's along with a black leather do-rag. I had not seen him in years. He looked fit, non-cancerous for certain, so I asked him who he had come there to support.

He glanced down at his shirt and said, "For myself, bud! I am here to gain inspiration from folks like you as I battle my recently diagnosed prostate cancer." He waved his well-muscled arm about at the milling crowd and then said, "Isn't this comradery *great*? It makes me feel almost *glad* to have gotten cancer!"

"Well," I responded, appraising his sculpted physique, "There doesn't appear to be anything *prostrate* about you! You appear to be in impressive shape, nothing like I looked while battling my salivary-gland cancer with chemo. Why, you even look *tan*!"

"Aw—that's probably from the radiation treatment," he chuckled, whapping my back so forcefully that I nearly fell forward.

"Ah, so that explains your vim and vigor—you avoided the ravages of chemo. But, then, why the do-rag?" (I asked because chemo causes total hair loss but radiation treatment does not.)

He grinned and lifted his do-rag to reveal an advanced but apparently natural pattern of balding up there and said, "Over the past ten years, I found myself using increasingly bizarre hairstyles, even trying a hairpiece or two, to conceal my growing baldness. Once I got cancer, I noticed how many cancer warriors wear do-rags, so—*why not*?"

He smiled, showing big bright teeth, and he pumped his fist in the aromatic air, glanced at my tee-shirt, and added, "So you beat your cancer, eh? 'Still ticking,' indeed! *Woo-hoo*!"

Then he punched some pain into my shoulder.

"Yea, sure," I replied: "Woo-hoo."

I made a fist of my own, but it dangled by my side. I simply could not share his enthusiasm at that moment.

"You look to have come through it in *fine* shape," he said, somewhat less sincerely, I thought. Winking, he added, "I should use you as a role model! You can't let cancer treatment get you down! My radiation treatments do burn my ass some, but I always go for gumption-restoring brewskis afterwards. Frankly, I'm about to head downtown to do just that! Want to come along?"

"Um—well—sounds good, Jer, but I think I'd better pass."

"What? Are you *still ticking* or what, my man? Matter of fact, why don't you get one of those 'cancer sucks' shirts over there at that stand with long lines? They're a huge help at meeting babes! Go get you one, and then let's go!"

He pounded my back again, leading to a brief coughing fit.

Upon recovery, I said, "Well Jer, I gotta get home soon for my evening meds, which do not mix well with alcohol."

I did not *actually* need to take them until much later, but I did *not* feel like bar-hopping with this nauseatingly upbeat dude.

"*Heart* meds?" he asked, incredulously.

I nodded, glancing down at my shirt, hoping it now would make better sense for him; but in case it didn't, I added, "My chemo treatments gave me congestive heart failure. Some joke, huh?"

"I'll say! What kind of a wimpy-ass condition is *that*?" He asked, shaking his s head in disappointment; and I did not see his big whitened teeth again. I did however soon hear this: "Well bud, I gotta run! Good luck with your, uh, little problem!"

Off he scurried, glancing all about.

Walking off to find Reg, I again thought, *I'd rather have cancer*. Next, I saw all of the recently-lit candles that circled the track that we had walked around—candles lit for those yet fighting cancer and for those who had lost their fights. I contemplated it for quite a while. At last, I kicked myself in the ass, or tried to—but I discovered that, technically, it was impossible to do so, at least for me.

Shortly after that failed attempt, I felt a toe-tap on my booty. I turned, and there stood Reg, who smilingly said, "Whatever you needed that for, you're welcome! I'm ready to cruise if you are. Plus, I just learned that a little wine is great for your heart!"

So, off we went.

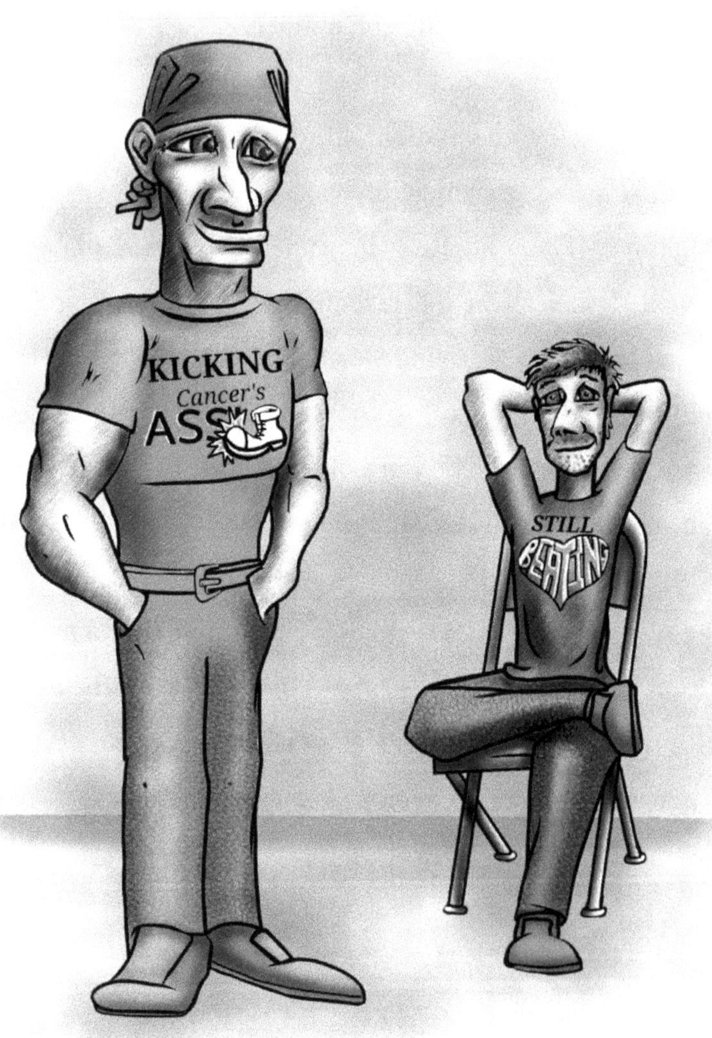
KICKING
Cancer's
ASS
STILL
BEATING

CHAPTER THREE

OR—JUST WHAT THE DOCTOR ORDERED?

A pessimist sees the difficulty in every opportunity; an optimist sees the opportunity in every difficulty. ~ Winston Churchill

No, dealing with CHF will never bestow the glamour and excitement of brawling with cancer. Still, it need not be all bad; and I needed to find some goodness in it. That would start with my cardiologist's orders regarding diet, exercise, and lifestyle: "Stay in shape!" he bellows; "Avoid stress," he murmurs.

I already felt that those were fine and worthy goals. Now I had a doctor's excuse to *always* do what I had previously done only when I could. Maybe this heart situation could lead to an improved lifestyle …

Chemo had kept me weak and overly thin, but my strength and appetite had been growing back, strength more slowly because at first I had been *afraid* of exercising's potential strain on my damaged heart. My second visit to my heart doc had recently changed that: Besides advising me to stay in shape, he had elaborated, "Do it, but just don't overdo it!" There is that moderation deal again!

Before cancer, I had tried to stay in shape to feel and look good; now I needed to stay in shape to *stay alive*. Very importantly for now, though, I would not *stress* about it. My heart doc always orders me to avoid stress, to take it easy. "Man," I tell him, "I've been trying to take it easy my whole life—but that's *not* easy!"

He tells me that in stressful situations my body releases "stress hormones" that could actually trigger a heart attack with my compromised ticker. Smiling as if joking, he also tells me that a humorous lifestyle possibly reduces the chances of such a stress-related heart attack. *Bingo*! People have always seemed to find my lifestyle humorous, even when I found it stressful. Maybe I should look at my life from *their* point of view?

I was about to vent on stressful things such as #/>^*%# childproof packaging that only a child can open, but I found it too stressful. Avoid such packaging! Bribe your three-year-old to open them!

Harder to avoid are those high-strung humans whose neck veins bulge and whose voices crack as they jab their fingers and ceaselessly rant about politics, economics, and society. You know the type—not only is the glass half-empty, but it is also polluted and indicative of moral decay and social disease. Their own hearts are typically strong; otherwise, they would have dropped dead of stress in their youth. Instead, their long-lived purpose is to give stress-caused heart-attacks to otherwise happy-go-lucky types like you and me. Let's call them "heart-attackers."

Although I am doing fairly well at avoiding these heart-attackers, a number of them are related to me, making total avoidance impossible. Take my Uncle—um, let's just call him "Uncle Hawkeyes." He is one of those people who, instead of talking with you, talks *at* you, at least when he is not shrieking at you. Like with most heart-attackers, you must carefully choose your topics; even discussing the weather can produce a socio-political tirade—greenhouse gases, for example.

Uncle Hawkeyes recently drove me to an out-of-town doctor's appointment (these heart-attackers are not *all* bad). Before he could switch on the outburst-rousing talk-radio that he normally listens to, I chose the most neutral conversation subject I could think of: the homemade veggie soup that "Aunt Dove-eyes" had graciously served us for lunch.

"So how about that veggie soup? *Yummy*, huh?"

I noticed his hawkish eyes shift back and forth in the rear-view mirror. His forehead veins throbbed; his breathing quickened. Uh-oh . . .

At least we paid for those vegetables with our own hard-earned money," he began, "not like the weasels that use food stamps paid for by—*stolen* from—our taxes."

Glancing daggers at moneyless me, he continued, "Speaking of hard-earned money, can you believe the price of vegetables and everything else at grocery stores these days?"

"Well, at least they're *fresh*," I cheerfully commented.

"Fresh? How could they be fresh coming from Mexico the way that most of them do?"

He jabbed a finger against the dashboard. "And who knows what kinds of preservatives keep them *supposedly* 'fresh'? Meanwhile, this is just one more way that Mexicans take American jobs!"

"Yea, those *damn* Mexicans" I agreeably agreed, patting his hunched shoulder while silently reminiscing about some Senoritas I have known.

"Still, even then the prices are astronomically high! You want to know why?"

"Um—false profits?"

"Nope, gas prices! Not to mention the ongoing war in the Middle East . . . "

And so he rambled forth, in the next ten minutes educating me on terrorism, national security, environmental damage, the national debt, and what *needs* done regarding each of them.

Although I smiled at this amazing romp through thorny topics, I also felt my chest tighten as, after a brief pause, he again opened his venom-spewing mouth.

"Hey, Unc," I interposed, "This type of talk is stressing me out, and my cardiologist *insists* that I avoid stress. How about some music instead—or at least some pleasant talk?"

Rather than launching into a new harangue against the health care situation as I feared he would, he said, "Oh," in a much softer voice as his shoulders un-hunched and his veins diminished. "Well then—how *about* that veggie soup?"

So, for my health, I need to avoid stressful heart-attackers like Uncle Hawkeyes; and that I will gladly do—this is just what the doctor ordered. Just as important for my new stress-free lifestyle, I decided I should also minimize the presence in my life of those mini-Martians who stress me out by breaking my things, eating my sweets, and jabbering at me all at the same time. Kids do warm my heart, which must be good for it, but they also frequently frazzle my nerves, which must be bad for it.

Early on, with my writing "career" off to a slow start (not that it has ever attained high speed), babysitting became a second career, an income-booster; although I no longer need that boost, the label of "great babysitter" has stuck, presumably to my behind, next to the sticker that says, "sucker!" Some people pack their troubles off to daycare; the others send them to me. The hitch is that true kids have always viewed me as a slightly wrinkled big kid. I keep some toys for them, but it sometimes seems that *I* am their favorite toy. No problem—at least not until I am officially sitting them.

Me: "Time for bed!"

They: "Tag! You're it!"

I do not need such stress, cannot allow it with this disquieting new heart issue. Plus, I *hate* tag! Besides that, while contemplating this midget-manufactured stress, clenching my fists and grinding my false teeth, I noticed this cautionary label on my heart-med bottle:

"KEEP AWAY FROM CHILDREN"

That seems clear enough to me! I *must* keep away from kids, especially in the trouble-fraught zone of babysitting.

I suppose babysitting for family is still okay, at least in a limited way. After all, I have a genetic stake in those kids. Besides, if necessary I can beat them into submission and nobody will call the cops. I just should not damage them *genetically.*

What I can no longer tolerate is being at the babysitting beck-and-call of non-relatives. I have no genetic stake in their imps—in fact, genetically-speaking I may have a stake in *eliminating* them, *theoretically speaking*, of course

Either way, it is best that I no longer sit for these non-relatives. . . . I made this clear when I received a typical sitting request the other day from my third cousin's best friend's sister-in-law.

She got right to it: "You doin' anything tomorrow night?"

"Just trying to write a book, that's all, not much," I warily answered.

"Oh, *good*! You want to watch the kids then?"

I counted to three, took several deep breaths, fleetingly considered a quick trip to the liquor store, and said, "Too bad you can't babysit this book I'm writing. *Trying* to write."

"Oh, you're still *funny*, I see. That's why my kids love you."

"Yea, they're funny, too," I responded, trying to scare her off. "Since they only recently learned to walk and talk, I always feel bad about telling them to sit down and shut up."

She sounded a bit more hesitant, saying, "Oh—you're trying to be funny again, *right*? So, can you sit them or not?"

I briefly considered telling her I had been thinking about registering as a sex offender—word would quickly spread among the babysitter-needy crowd . . . but since I could not then, under those heart meds, sexually offend even a porno queen, I instead said what I should have at the start: "No, I can't."

Disbelief in her voice, she asked, "Why not?"

Gazing at my heart-med bottle, I smilingly said, "Sorry, doctor's orders!" Then I added, "Spread the word!"

If cancer ever takes me down, I will go down fighting. If heart failure takes me down, it will likely catch me in my recently installed hammock—I'll go down daydreaming.

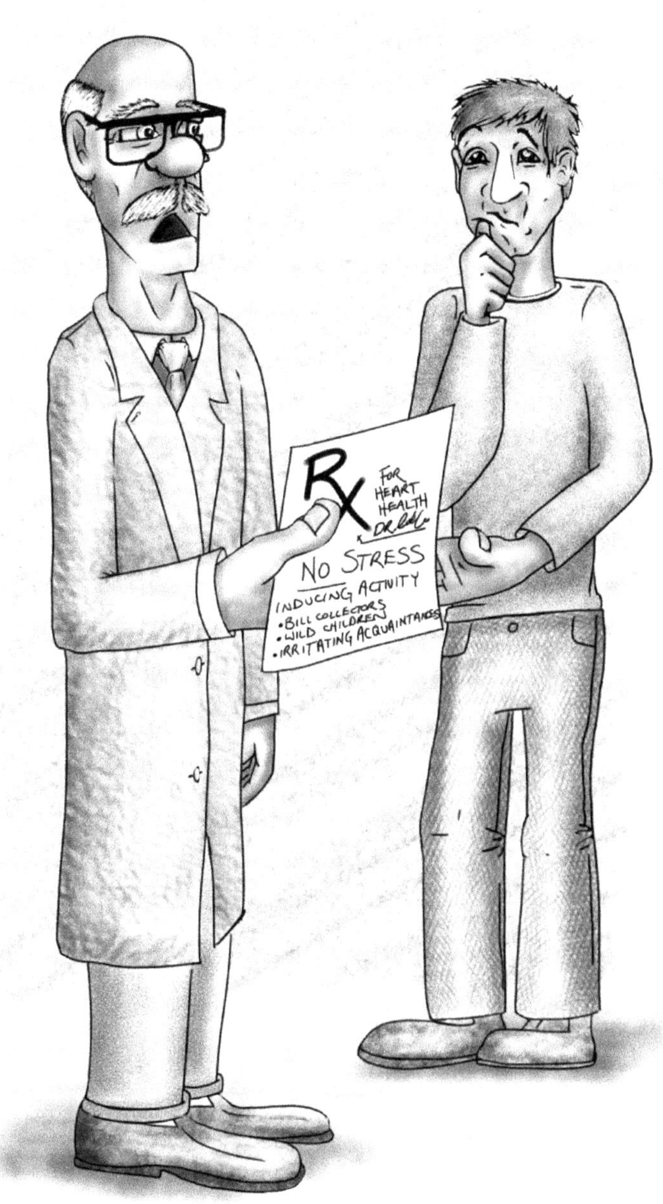
RX
FOR
HEART
HEALTH
NO STRESS
INDUCING ACTIVITY
•BILL COLLECTORS
•WILD CHILDREN
•IRRITATING ACQUAINTANCES

CHAPTER FOUR

THE HEART-ATTACK ALL-STARS

Be not afraid of greatness; some are born great, others achieve greatness, and others have greatness thrust upon them.
~ William Shakespeare

Had I allowed the imps to cause me a heart attack, this would have been natural and commonplace. Others, however, have had far more exciting heart attack experiences—these are the All-Stars in the World of Heart Attacks.

When young and overconfident, thinking I had a destiny as a pro baseball player, I studied the habits and histories of the star players. Years later, and still confident, thinking I had a destiny as a writer, I studied the personal habits and histories of the great writers—boy, could they drink! Now that my true destiny seemingly is to have a heart attack, I recently sought out the habits, the histories, the heart-stopping achievements of the cardiac-arrested mega-stars—those who went out in style and with pizzazz. So grab a greasy pizza-burger or pop some buttery popcorn and have a seat!

We will first look at those who went out on top, at the pinnacles of success; and while many people at other types of pinnacles might say, "I thought I'd died and gone to heaven," these All-Stars actually *did* die and go to, presumably, heaven.

I have known many bowlers—people who bowl for "sport"—and so I know how hard it is to bowl a perfect game of 300. Our first All-Star, Donald Doanne, who lived and died in Michigan (where bowling, *not* college football, is the State Sport) always knew how hard it is, too; because after bowling for 45 years, he had *never* achieved a *perfect* game.

Then, one October night, perhaps trying to somehow counter-balance the deficiencies of Michigan football, he finally did it! When the pins of the final strike had all scattered and disappeared into the depths, Don pumped a fist as his teammates surrounded him and slapped his broad back—a perfect game! Shortly after, his heart stopped the party by stopping its beating; and Don collapsed, perfectly dead, downed in a blaze of glory.

Hearing of this bittersweet Michigan "sports" tale, I telephoned the football coach of the Michigan Wolverines.

"Coach ~~Hoke~~ Harbaugh," I said, "In honor of the recently downed Michigan sportsman, Don Doanne, why don't you rename your team the 'Michigan Bowlers?' It would furnish your team *and* their fans with precisely the dignity that they deserve."

I cannot in this family-oriented book, fully quote his reply; but I can tell you that at the end of it was, "Go to hell." Don, who did *not* go there, is likely in the other place right now, asking Jesus if he would care for a game of bowling on water.

Odds are that All-Star #2, Donald Peters, went in the same upward direction on his Big Day. From there, he likely sent messages to his widow telling her to never throw away a lottery ticket without first checking its numbers against the winning numbers.

You see, on the last day of his life, Donald stopped at a local store and purchased lottery tickets for himself and for his wife of 59 years, Charlotte. Shortly after returning from the store, while working in his yard he had the 'Big One.' This in itself hardly makes him an All-Star. (Countless people have had heart attacks while working—which is why I avoid it.)

What makes Mr. Peters an All-Star is this: several months later, right after contemplating throwing them away, Widow Peters *finally* checked those lottery tickets' numbers—she had a winner, six million dollars' worth. *That* makes Donald one of our All-Stars.

Despite her heaven-sent wealth, 78-year-old Charlotte announced that she had no plans to move out of her trailer park.

So, we can imagine angelic All-Star Donald at the edge of a heavenly cloud, shouting down at her, "Move out of that damn trailer before you give me *another* heart attack!"

Humor is allegedly beneficial for heart health. Nevertheless, our next two All-Stars went out amidst laughter—which makes them All-Stars, although dead ones at that. If more people died laughing, maybe death would not have such a bad reputation; then again, laughter's reputation may take a hit.

Out Heart-Attack All-Star #3 ~~is~~ was from England. These ~~are~~ were, after all, *international* stars. English speaking people often say, "I thought I'd die laughing." Well, Alex Mitchell ~~thinks~~ thought words are cheap—a bricklayer, he ~~is~~ was a man of action.

His Big Last Moments came while watching a British TV comedy, *The Goodies*. After 25 continuous minutes of laughing at The Goodies, he had 'The Big One' and *literally* died laughing, which makes him one of our stars.

Alex's widow Nessie later wrote to the TV show's stars and actually *thanked* them for making his last moments so enjoyable, even though he had not bought a winning lottery ticket earlier in the day. He did, however, go out in style; and I find it inspirational. We come into the world crying; to leave it laughing signals *progress*.

Unconfirmed reports report that Alex currently spends *his* time laughing at All-Star Donald Peters as he peers over the edge of their heavenly cloud and shouts for his widow to sell or give away that damn trailer.

Or—perhaps he's actually laughing up there at Dick Shawn, our next Heart-Attack All-Star. Shawn ~~is~~ was the *truly* funny one among our stars, an accomplished comic-actor and stand-up comedian.

He had not always sought fame as a comedian; as a young man, he had instead aimed for fame as a professional baseball player; but getting drafted for the Vietnam War cut that dream short. Like I had done, he ultimately gave up his baseball dream to become a jokester.

He had his Big One while performing onstage in San Diego. Reports varied on what his routine was just prior to the attack—either politicians lying down on the job or nuclear war—but either way it seemed like part of the act when he lay down face-first onstage and did not move.

And he did not move.

Again, for a while it seemed like part of his act. The audience watched, smiling; and some even started commenting—one sit-down comedian yelled, "Take his wallet!"

And he did not move.

Finally, a stagehand came onstage, not to take Shawn's wallet, but to take his pulse; and then he shouted this dramatic question: "Is there a doctor in the house?"

San Diego happens to have nearly as many doctors as it has the lawyers who sue them, and so a doctor soon came onstage while countless lawyers watched in the wings.

And he did not move.

At this point, still thinking it all an act, some of the audience got rude, even labeling it as a *distasteful* routine.

It has been a long time since I lived in San Diego, and I do not know just how outrageous their political correctness standards are these days. However, my guess is that if the audience thought Shawn (I love it when last names are like first names) was pretending to be a dead republican, *that* would have been okay, maybe even hilarious, at least to the San Diego Democrats.

Meanwhile, resuscitation efforts failed, effectively shutting up the rude ones and sending up to Heaven our Heart-Attack All-Star #4: Dick Shawn, a stand-up guy even when he lay down. Unconfirmed reports confirm that Shawn makes a heavenly living by telling jokes about the devil and about Michigan football.

Like Shawn, Heart-Attack All-Star #5 was already famous when he too died on stage, leaving behind this unspoken message: *be careful what you brag about*!

Skipping childhood, James Rodale spent his adult life as founder and CEO of Rodale Press, publishers of a zillion books and magazines on living healthily. Many of these publications emphasize that one could, through right living, live for a very long time or even longer than that—one recent Rodale Press title is *Transcend: Nine Steps to Living Well Forever*.

At age 72, Rodale himself was somewhat short of forever when he was interviewed on-tape for a never-aired segment of old-time TV's *The Dick Cavett Show*.

During that interview, the elderly, yet seemingly robust Rodale bragged thusly: "I'm in such good health that I fell down a long flight of stairs yesterday and laughed all the way."

I know more than a few drunks who could make similar claims, so I am not that impressed.

Rodale also declared that "I'm going to live to be 100 unless I'm run down by some sugar-crazed taxi-driver."

Note that he said this at a time when sugar was the major urban narcotic. Note also that, as Rodale was a zillionaire, he probably rode limousines, not taxis, so he would likely never have actually spied any taxi drivers sniffing, smoking or injecting sugar.

While still in the interview chair, Rodale suddenly stopped boasting and slumped down. Host Cavett leaned over and asked, "Are we boring you, Mr. Rodale?"

Nope, he was not bored; he was dead. Heart-Attack All-Star James Rodale—he talked a good game, albeit a shorter one than he had planned. We hear that he spends his heavenly time lecturing to God on how, by living right, He could live forever.

Our Heart-Attack All-Star #6, Clayton Lockett, is a star not because he went out on top or onstage, but because his heart attack beat 'The Man.'

You see, the state of Oklahoma (aka, 'The Man') sought to execute Clayton via the lethal injection of three drugs, given one by one, the third one meant to stop his heart. Perhaps sensing the danger, or maybe just to piss off 'The Man,' Clayton's heart stopped beating *before* that third drug. This *definitely* did piss off 'The Man!'

When his heart stopped on its own, with no help from 'The Man,' this *proved* that Clayton had not been a totally *heartless* criminal. Unimpressed, 'The Man' called a doctor and drew the curtains to the execution room's viewing gallery *so that spectators who had come to watch the execution could not watch the "horrible thing to witness."* We Heart-Attack connoisseurs call an execution a horrible thing to witness; however, we call *that* heart attack "a splendid and awesome performance."

It also gave otherwise bored-stiff reporters plenty of material to make a 'Big Deal' out of . . . **"BOTCHED EXECUTION"** appeared in all headlines. (What they call a botched execution, we—while thumbing our noses at 'The Man'—call an All-Star worthy Heart Attack. What timing!)

Unconfirmed reports report that, to avoid such botching in the future, 'The Man' will henceforth serve only heart-healthy final meals so that condemned inmates will survive long enough to be properly killed not by 'The Lord,' but by 'The Man.'

Heart-Attack All-Star Cayton Lockett: his heart stopped beating, not when it was told to stop beating, but when it felt like it. Nonetheless, up in heaven Clayton is reportedly nowhere to be found.

Our *seventh* and *final* Heart-Attack All-Star is/was not *only* a Star, but was also the charter member of our planned Heart Attack Hall of Fame. Fifty-Two year old John Alleman was a daily customer at, a spokesman for, and had his 'Big One' outside of the Las Vegas *Heart Attack Grille*—an ideal location for our Hall of Fame. I actually telephoned the hearty restaurant's manager, Jon Basso, and proposed placing our Heart-Attack Hall of Fame there. He laughed. After I sternly informed him that I ~~was~~ am serious, he then said a few things that, since this is not Vegas but a PG-rated publication, I cannot repeat.

This restaurant, with an old ambulance out front, has a hospital theme, calling its scantily clad young waitresses "nurses," its customers "patients," and its meal-orders "prescriptions." Their specialty, "Bypass Burgers," range from a mere half-pounder "Single Bypass" to a two-pounder "Quadruple Bypass" burger; with five slices of greasy bacon per 8-ounce patty, the Quadrupal Bypass Burger gets twenty slices. If you are determined to join the late Mr. Alleman in our Heart-Attack Hall-of-Fame, you might also fill up on

"Flatliner Fries" fried in *pure* lard and wash it all down with a cola, beer, tequila or (best yet) a thick "Butter-fat Shake."

Customers who finish a Triple- or Quadruple-Bypass Burger get rewarded by being placed in a wheelchair and wheeled out to their vehicle by a busty personal "nurse." On the other cheek, those who fail to finish their heart-stopping meal get playfully paddled by their undoubtedly lascivious "nurse"—I hope they use a large paddle, because I think we are talking big buttocks!

So, this is the environment that All-Star John Alleman daily chose to frequent—an environment where heart-attacks had previously happened, usually involving burgers, liquor, and cigarettes. He had his 'Big One' at the bus-stop outside of his favorite place, the Heart Attack Grille, an end *so poetic* that we—or at least *I*—can contemplate it only in awe.

Unreported confirmations hint that John spends his time Up There searching for Noah, whom he respectfully, yet hungrily, *suspects* has hidden the heavenly cows. Regardless, here on earth John died as he had lived, a fine way to go. For that, we name him Heart-Attack Hall-of-Famer #1.

And ~~anxiously~~ relaxingly await all challengers …

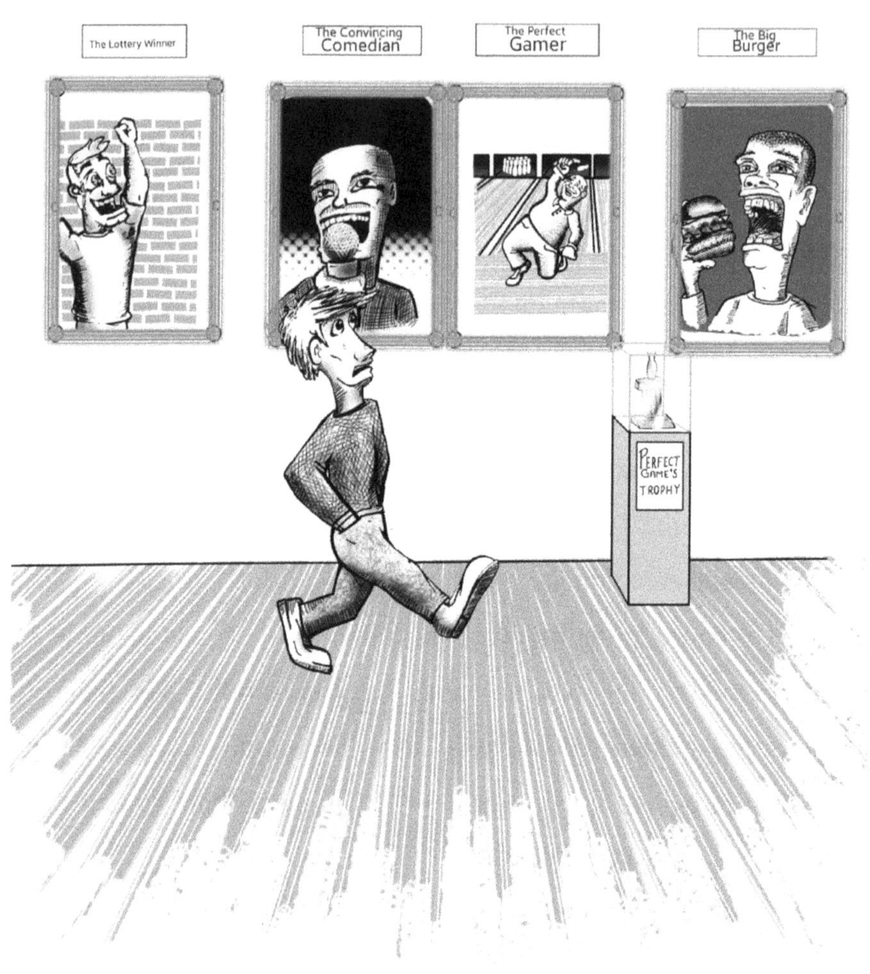
The Lottery Winner
The Convincing Comedian
The Perfect Gamer
The Big Burger
PERFECT GAME'S TROPHY

CHAPTER FIVE

HEARTS DON'T BEAT LIKE THEY USED TO

Keep a green tree in your heart, and perhaps a singing bird will come. ~ Chinese proverb

Our hearts are beating when we are born, and they beat until we die—when hearts stop, life stops quickly. I say, "*Go hearts, go*!"

Having recently learned about some of the colorful characters of the heart, I now wished to learn some Heart History. So, I went to visit one whose heart has beat longer than about anyone's—my great-great Aunt Rose, who, I am sure, *never* patronized the Heart Attack Grille.

Aunt Rose met me at the front door, early afternoon on a recent weekday.

The very old lady looked good, and I said so: "You're looking youthful today, auntie!"

"Oh, I *am* young at heart," she replied, "but I am somewhat older in other places."

"I'll say," I thought-not-said, following her wobbly willowy figure into the sitting room.

She seemed ancient when I was a young kid. Back then my mother would sometimes tell us that Aunt Rose used to babysit baby Jesus. Other times she said that Aunt Rose had been the waitress at the Last Supper—and we believed it!

As Aunt Rose showed me to a comfy chair, she asked, "You been sleeping okay?"

"Good enough," I replied as the stuffed chair half-swallowed me.

"So, you probably don't pull anymore all-nighters—*do you*?"

"Nope, Auntie. An 'all-nighter' to me these days means not having to get up to pee!"

"Oh!" She smiled. "Well, you probably go to bed hoping you'll feel okay when you wake up. I go to bed hoping just to wake up! How would you like a beer? I'm getting me one."

"It's kind of early," I told her, pleasantly enough, I thought.

"It's five o'clock somewhere," she snapped. "You used to be a lot more fun when you had cancer, you know. Well, what *would* you like to drink?"

"Um—a diet cola?"

"Yech! That stuff will give you *cancer*!" Aunt Rose quipped,

"Maybe," I admitted, "but it's good for the heart—or, at least better than beer."

Shaking her grey old head, she disappeared into the kitchen, soon returning with a 12-ounce diet cola for me and a 24-ounce beer for herself.

"The doctor told me one beer per day" she announced, settling into her rocker. "Of course, she did *not say* how many per night!" She cackled, rocked, and sipped.

"Um—do you drink much beer?" I asked, to start our conversation. but I was interested, too; because I had known her to drink her own homemade brandy, but *never* canned beer.

"Not usually," she said, "because it brings on that old urge to smoke."

"I—I didn't know you used to smoke!"

"Yep, but I quit cold-turkey one day, hopefully early enough to help my longevity."

I smiled—if she was a hundred, she was a hundred and a day.

"How long ago did you quit?" I asked, thinking it would have been long before my birth.

"Oh, about ten years ago," she said, rocking, sipping.

I was about to comment on that when her old rotary-dial land-line phone rang back in the kitchen. Creaking and crackling, she rose and headed that way.

Before long, I heard snippets of her speaking sharply into the phone "No, no *no!* . . . What did you say to me? . . . I told the last jerk who called *not* to call again!"

I was about to go see if I should get involved, when I heard, "If you *do* come here, I have a baseball bat just for you right inside my door!"

I glanced that way and saw—yes, a dinged old club-sized one—as I heard the classical sound of a phone *slamming* down.

Aunt Rose reappeared, taking a healthy swig of beer as she snapped and popped back into her rocker, saying, "Selling burial plots! Imagine! And, here I've already had one for, what? About 60 years now! Right beside my first husband Albert, the father of my children."

I remembered an interesting story about the great-great uncle that I never knew, Uncle Albert.

"Dad told me that Albert used to play semi-pro baseball as a switch *pitcher.* He said he'd take two gloves to the mound, pitching left-handed to lefties and right-handed to righties," I said, reminicing a bit.

"Yes, yes, and after his playing years, for as long as he lasted, which was not long, you'd find him summer nights under our backyard oak tree listening to radio broadcasts of the Indians of Cleveland," Aunt Rose then replied with a far off look in her eyes.

Aunt Rose had outlived several husbands. I knew more about Albert than about the others, all before my time.

"He must have passed fairly young. . . What from?" I asked, as she smiled.

"'Passed' is something one does in the bathroom, hopefully." she said. "He *died* at age forty-one, after fitting a hundred years of ball-playing and drinking into those years. Died of, yes, a heart attack. He had a bum-ticker—like I hear you do. Thing is, *he* never let it slow *him* down."

She took another swig of beer.

I sipped my diet cola and leaned forward.

"My cardiologist tells me that my heart meds—a beta blocker and an ACE inhibitor—keep me alive. Those weren't around back then, I guess."

"*Back then*? Well, I guess by now you know that I never actually babysat the little Lord Jesus?"

Another full smile—she had in her lower dental plate this day—and another swig of beer.

"No, not *those* medicines," she continued after a tiny, ladylike belch. "Heart surgery had been around for a couple decades, the technology improving all the time—not that Albert and I could afford *that*. Heart disease had been announced as the number one killer in the country about a month before Albert died from it. Could have fooled us!"

She paused and momentarily shut her eyes.

"He died with a half-empty bottle of scotch whiskey under his bed—I guess that must've been the number two killer. Since then, there have been many heart transplants, ongoing attempts at mechanical hearts . . ."

"*That* sounds so, um, cold hearted, so robotic," I interjected. "I'll take my natural, organic heart any day, flaws and all!"

"Oh," she nodded, "And I suppose you believe that your heart is the center of yourself, of love and emotions, the place where your soul might reside?"

"Well—I don't know about all *that*."

"Here," she said, creaking up, turning toward the tall bookshelves behind her, "I've got a book for you."

After fingering through the dusty stacks, she emerged with a paperback, which she handed to me. Its title was *A Change of Heart*.

"Modern medicine, and the very concept of mechanical hearts, tells us to view the heart as a mere pump. This book is by a lady who received a transplanted real heart and then took on the personality traits of the heart donor—it calls that medical view into question." She sat back down, seemingly winded.

"Hmm—well, thanks," I said, wondering if I might actually read it—I had been reading mysteries almost exclusively, lately.

"Scientists sure have learned a lot in my time," Aunt Rose continued, "hut one guesses that they will never know everything, that some things will remain a *mystery.*"

"I *love* mysteries!" I blurted, and then more calmly added, "Like how astronomers can calculate backwards to the Big Bang—all the way back to within a microsecond of it, describing how the universe has expanded ever since, but they can get no further back to the very beginning, the creation of the universe, than that microsecond."

"Yes, but they—not just astronomers, scientists—*they* can tell us the heart is simply a collection of muscles, valves, and vessels," she said, and swigged.

"Also that the body is a collection of chemicals valued at about ten bucks," I added, and sipped.

"That reminds me of a PBS science program I recently watched," said Aunt Rose, rocking. "A whole panel of scientists from different disciplines—biology, chemistry, whatnot—described in great detail the precise conditions under which life must have first begun eons ago."

She paused, emptied her beer, and continued. "They even had an image of an ancient tide pool of the type in which it might have happened. They *knew* the exact temperature, the strict combination of chemicals, the precise salinity and oxygen levels of the water, all supposedly energized by a bolt of lightning—*everything*, according to them, necessary for life to emerge from the un-life."

"Wow," I said, "Did they, you know, actually create life by recreating those conditions?" I asked, thinking surely I would have heard if they had succeeded.

"Nope, nephew. I watched and waited, but those renowned scientists who *knew*, just *knew* everything about the requirements of life and its beginning, they *never*, not one, said that in their laboratory simulations they had *themselves* created actual life, even in its *simplest* form. *That* remains a mystery—and this old lady guesses it will stay one."

She smiled, rocked a little, and then her ancient eyelids drooped down.

"Aunt Rose! You want to lay down for a nap?" I asked, as leaned down and kissed her surprisingly smooth forehead.

Eyes completely closed now, she gently rocked and softly said, "No, I'm good right here. You know your way out, right? Don't forget your book."

Clutching the book, I silently let myself out—the heavy door creaked just like great-great Aunt Rose's knees …

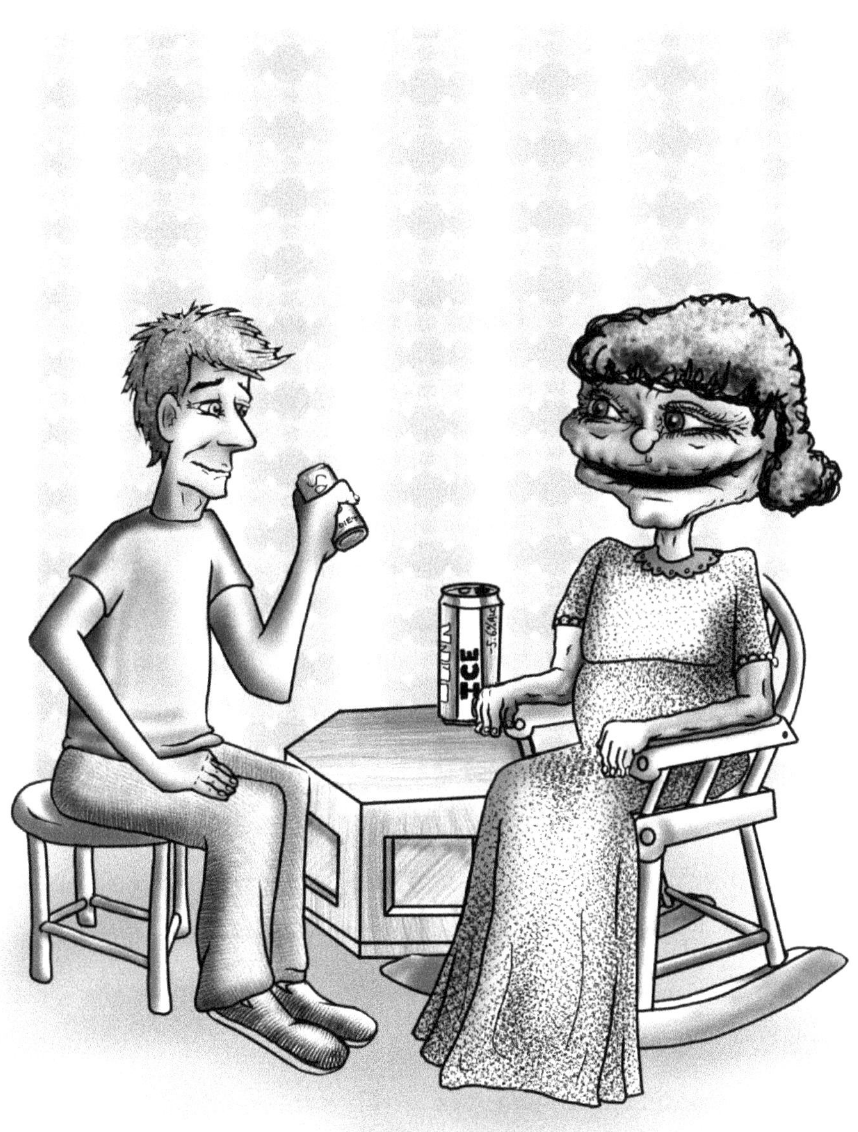
ICE

CHAPTER SIX

ONE MEDIUM HEART, WITH A SIDE-ORDER OF PERSONALITY

The heart has reasons that reason cannot know.
~ Blaise Pascal

Just a few nights later, I began to read the book that Aunt Rose had lent me, *A Change of Heart* by Claire Sylvia—*ah*, another last name that sounds like a first name! I soon discovered that, like the novels I had recently been reading, this autobiographical book by a heart-transplant recipient concerned a *mystery*: when someone receives a heart from someone else, do they receive more than a specialized pump? Do they also gain personality traits of the (necessarily deceased) heart-donor?

According to Sylvia, yes—with a transplanted heart you do get some of the donor's personality, some of their history. If this is true, and true for other organs too, I am taking "liver" off of my donor card—it has too many memories that I would rather keep to myself!

Some "medical people" actually have a "scientific" theory to account for this, and they call it "cellular memory." To put this theory into layman's and laywoman's (henceforth known as laypersons) terms, it means that individual cells have memories that help them to function; when someone receives someone else's organs, consisting of cells, they would also receive those memories.

Not all "medical people," and not many medical *doctors*, accept this theory. I was, nonetheless, troubled by imagined images of my elderly neighbor, who has received a pig's heart valve, literally rooting through my garbage; consequently, I conducted a very brief survey of doctors—in short, I asked my own cardiologist what he thinks of "cellular memory." He respectfully termed it, "El bunko. Totally stinkarooni!"

Unable to just blindly accept such technical jargon, I decided to *personally* investigate plainly reported reports of heart transplant patients whose post-transplant experiences prove otherwise. I started by flipping to Chapter Two of Sylvia's book …

Way back in 1988, middle-aged Claire Sylvia, a fully feminine professional dancer/choreographer, received a heart from a younger man who had very recently died in a motorcycle accident, making him a manly man, albeit a dead one. Now, she did *not* report *this* in her book; but I imagine that when she appeared in a leather biker-babe outfit in the hospital gift shop and asked the clerk where to find the hospital's tattoo parlor, this should have been a clue of changes to come.

Whether or not I have that scenario right, Sylvia *did* admit to the following trait-changes, which she later learned matched her late donor's habits: a health-food nut, she suddenly craved, purchased, and devoured nauseatingly greasy chicken nuggets of an unnamed fried-poultry franchise from hillbilly-land with a founder who looks like an intellectual Santa; she felt "different" when hugging (and perhaps groping, though she does not admit *that*) her female friends. Formerly a wine-sipper, she became a beer-guzzler; and she also lost the desire to cook—although not the desire to go out to eat.

She naturally connected these startling changes to her new heart that had formerly been owned by a motorcycling, nugget-gnawing, testosterone addled, beer-guzzling, non-cooking young man.

Could all of *this* evidence prove the controversial "cellular memory" theory? Scientists will say no, not by itself. We need a larger sample size. Unfortunately, not everyone who gets a heart transplant then writes a whole book about it, so I rolled up my sleeveless shirt and turned to the internet—what follows is what I found. . .

I found some *fascinating* case histories that mysteriously named no names. No problem! We will boldly name them as we go.

First, an unnamed girl who we will call "Shirley" received a heart from a ten-year-old murder victim we will call "Vic Jr." Shirley soon started to have dreams about the murder, including the place of the murder, the weapon used, the murderer's appearance, and even the clothes that he wore.

Her psychiatrist, who we will name "Doc," believed these dreams so strongly that he or she contacted the cops, who then located and arrested the child-killer, who we will call "the creep." For the murdered young heart-donor, this was better than revenge from the grave—it was instead from a youthful chest in which his heart beats on.

Nearly as dramatically, an 18-year-old boy that we will call "Tim" (we would have called him "Timmy" if he was 17 or younger) wrote songs and played music, recording a song titled "Danny, My Heart Is Yours," about dying and donating his heart. When he actually did die in a car crash, his young heart was transplanted into a total stranger—an 18-year-old girl named Danielle, who we will call "Danny." Upon hearing the aforementioned song, she knew the words prior to hearing them. Her new heart must have told her.

Moving right along, a young woman who was an auto accident victim (Let's call her "Vicki") gave—via doctors and other medical people, of course—her heart *and* lungs to a young grad student who we will call "Brad" since it rhymes with "grad."

Vicki was reportedly a lesbian, although I found no proof of this in any of the web-based lesbian movies that I diligently researched, seeking evidence.

Meanwhile, Brad-rhymes-with-grad, unaware of his heart-donor's inclinations, worried at first that getting a woman's heart would make him gay, and we do not mean "happy."

Brad was much relieved that he instead became a stud, or at least a much more sensitive heterosexual lover very attuned to his female lover's body and its needs; she (let's call her "Lucky") says, "He's a much better lover now."

However, Lucky also says Brad indulges in constant hugging, often carries a purse, and loves to go shopping, especially at malls.

So, Brad gets a new heart, and Lucky gets an upgraded boyfriend *and* new girlfriend all in the same person. That is why we call her "Lucky."

In case you are not yet convinced that something strange is going on here, we will now get more scientific and use *real* names, even though that is way less fun. It is furthermore none too scientific to use only "feel good" stories, so let's put on our "feel bad" glasses. Let's get 100% scientific, and let's examine the tragic case of Sonny Graham, whom we will call "Graham," as in 'graham cracker;' because the name "Sonny" is not dramatic enough for our purposes.

Sonny Graham and his second-hand heart are nevertheless both dead. What a hard-luck heart—that's twice! But, as we will see, when alive it was a *foolish* heart both times …

In 1995, suffering from congestive heart failure (like me, except for the suffering part) Graham received a heart transplanted from Terry Cotte, who had just shot himself, obviously *not* in the heart. The operation was a success, and all went well—for a while.

Then, in 1997 Graham met his benefactor's widow, Cheryl Watkins—a name she would keep throughout her multiple marriages, perhaps as a feminist gesture, perhaps to keep some *permanence*, something she never got nor gave in her relationships. (Why change a name only to change it again, and again, and again?) Since she likes her original name so much, we will call her none of the other names that come to mind, but we will call her "Cheryl."

Graham's new heart apparently had *not* learned from its past mistakes—it fell again for Cheryl, 30 years younger than Graham. When asked about meeting Cheryl for the first time, he said, "I felt I knew her for years." So, he must have felt like he had known her since he was her age.

The two were practically inseparable from the start. After that, Cheryl needed some time away to slowly separate from her third and fourth husbands, who did *not* commit suicide.

Possibly in need of a brain transplant in 2001, Graham divorced his steady, loyal, aging wife of thirty years to have Cheryl move in with him. His second-hand heart beat either excitedly or nervously. Three years later, he became her fifth husband.

Always a mover and shaker—he even has a football stadium named after him—Graham evidently had no spare time in which to investigate and learn that Cheryl had threatened to kill *all* of her previous husbands; one had even had a restraining order placed against her.

Whether or not she ever threatened to kill Graham, she did not have to kill him because . . . poetically on April first (2008), we *think* he killed himself, with a gun-blast to the neck—thus preserving that foolish heart, now a two-time loser.

Questions were raised about the highly suspicious so-called suicide; the investigation into possible murder lasted awhile but found no strong proof.

Yes, Cheryl was free again to not change her name; but it would not again be with that same doomed heart, which was buried with Graham. (Then again, perhaps the bride-transplant, not the heart-transplant, may have been the real issue?)

So call me "unscientific" if you want, but I propose that these cases prove that personality weirdness sometimes happens when hearts change chests.

Anyway, it is not even a question for the scientists. No, it is instead a question for the poets—and we plan to ask them about it, just as soon as they 'sober up.'

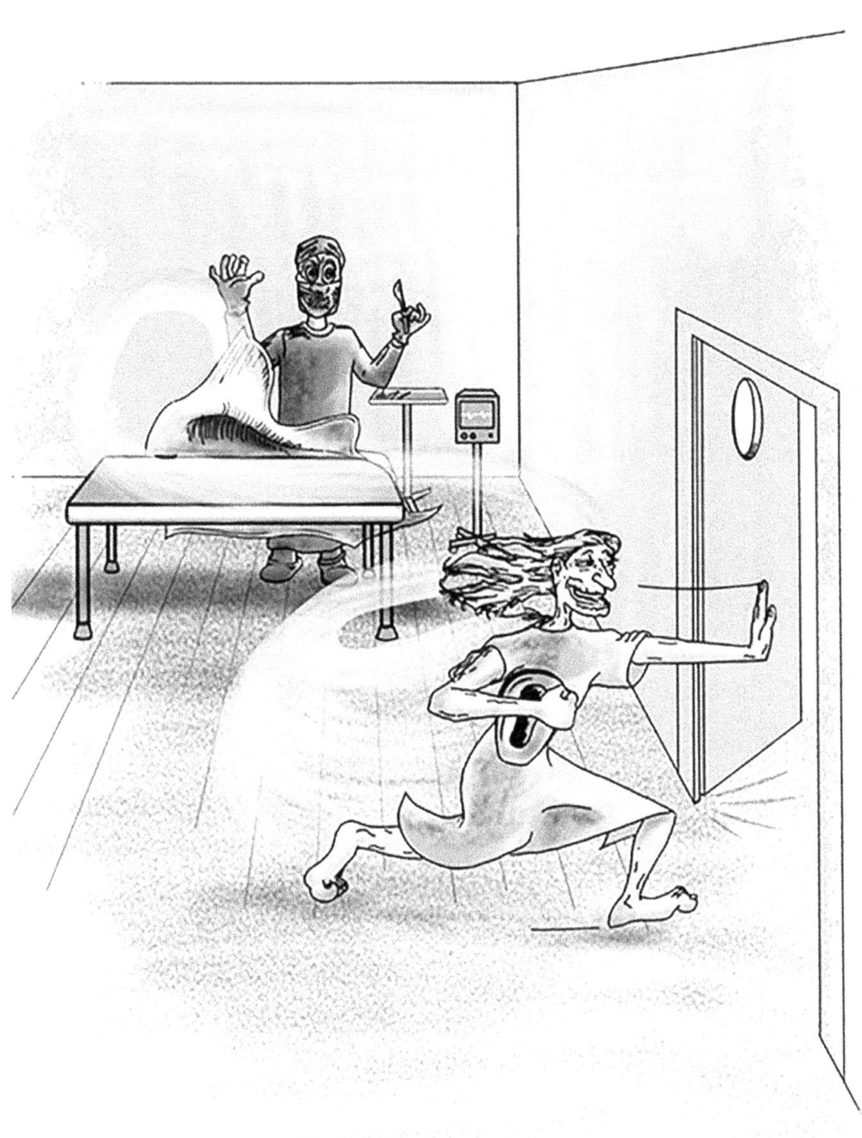

CHAPTER SEVEN

SEMI-HEAVY BREATHING

No matter how much cats fight, there always seem to be plenty of kittens. ~ Abraham Lincoln

Just as poets sometimes 'sober up,' it seemed to be time for me to 'get it up.' My curvy come-and-go girl. Karen (whom I call "Baby") had lately been intensifying her ~~demand~~ requests that I put my chemo-crippled past behind me and resume making love "like a regular guy"—only she means more regular than that! She urges me to once again become the love-making machine that I used to be. Rather than futilely argue that I never even was a machine, I must see what I can do about averting this pending love-nest crisis.

Heart issue and all, I still feel the same erotic urges that I felt at age 21—yes, I still urge after 21-year-old women (aka "Hotties"). Maybe "urge" is a bit strong—I "itch" or "hanker" toward them. Or, I *would*, but not since Karen came along, at least not while she is watching. I must have been tired of the pursuit of happiness when I entered into this "mature" relationship, one in which I often wear the apron in the family. I *did* let her know at our start who's the boss. I looked her straight in her arctic blue eyes and declared, "You're the boss!"

From that exulted position, she has taught me a lot. I now put the toilet seat down when done with my manly business. I no longer drink directly out of the milk or juice carton. I replace the toilet-paper roll over rather than under. I no longer clip my toenails in bed.

I have perfectly mastered these marks of civilization, these *gentlemanly* habits, but now she seems to want me to revert to animalism, *healthy* animalism! Newly a student of cardio-sexology, she tries to teach me of the cardio-health benefits of sex.

I tell her, "Karen, I don't want to drop dead of a heart attack while I'm on top of you!"

While waving a computer printout, she tells me, "The increased risk of a heart attack while doing it, *only* applies to those who *rarely* do it. I quote, 'Research suggests that having sex *at least* twice a week can help to *prevent* heart problems,' unquote."

Barely noticing the scintillating way that she placed a balled fist on each womanly hip and made her womanly lips pouty, I said, "Well okay then. Twice a week! We can do *that*."

"It says *at least* twice a week!"

"Well, then, okay, *at least* twice a week," I said. "Um— but how do you interpret *that*?"

"It means five or six times per week," she replied, and then burst into girlish giggles, and so I kissed her madly.

That led to, well, you *know* what that led to. Afterwards, I resisted saying, *one down and one to go!* Karen is, after all, a wonderfully inventive tigress in bed, always surprising me with the things we might do—this time, something with clothespins that I am too embarrassed to talk about here. She's so kinky, when she was born and the doctor slapped her butt, she tried to say, "Pinch me, too!"

Yes, but now, with my heart struggling, maybe even *failing*, we needed to reduce the kinkiness, less it puts a kink in my lifespan.

So, last week I had gotten her to agree to get rid of our wilder sex toys: sex rocks, pleasure tape, candy pants, a feather duster, a "Naughty Nurse Outfit," and all kinds of simpler sexy gizmos. Now, the only whip that remained in our bedroom would be whipped cream—preferably nonfat.

Karen, who had only wistfully agreed in principle to rid ourselves of these potentially heart-stopping stimulation-aids, now advanced a sole objection:

"You threw out *my* candy panties?" she pouted. "Out with the empty milk cartons and moldy bread and slimy soup cans? How *horrid*!"

"What'd you want me to do—throw a garage sale with that stuff? Reduced prices on jeans, sweaters, candy panties, and naughty nurse outfits?"

She smiled and returned to her web browsing. Finally, she announced, "Sex is the cause of only about 1% of heart attacks! What are you worried about?"

"About making it 1.1%!"

"Oh, be a man about it, *boy*," she said, again scanning her laptop screen, lightly humming to herself.

Then she said, "Listen to this: 'Attila the Hun won many battles in his lifetime, but he died of a heart attack on his wedding night.' How *romantic*!"

As I settled back on the couch with my new *Basket Weaving for Beginners* book, she scanned anew. "And—listen to this! Matthew McConaughey's dad died while making love to his wife, who said in her book that it was the best way for him to go—that she was *proud* of having such a husband, dying in her arms!"

"You'd think she'd be proud of having a man who stuck around a long time," I said. "He probably had a nice big life insurance policy. Well, I *don't. S*o you can forget that."

"That attitude figures! You're the type of guy who'd rather die in your *own* arms!"

This started a bit of a spat. Yes, I had some words with her, and she had some *paragraphs* with me. Not that I mind when Karen gets in the last word—it's a joy when she gets to her last word. But we were far from that!

Again pointing at her laptop, she said, almost diplomatically, "Maybe it's not *all* your fault. Those beta-blockers that you take more than double your chances of erectile dysfunction."

"Oh, *great,"* I responded. "The word 'failure' is already attached to my health; why not add 'dysfunction'? A *dysfunctional failure*—how nice! Tickets on sale to the freak show right here!"

"Don't despair," Karen urged in a cheerleading tone. "This article says it's okay to mix in Viagra with beta blockers. That way, you won't go when you come. It also says that heart attacks seldom occur during the exertion of sex because the exertion lasts a relatively short time. That means that you're *really* safe!"

"Oh yeah," I said, partly smiling. "Other studies show that men are more prone to heart attacks than are women because women are more prone to *giving* them."

"You don't say? Well, I'll just plan to sleep on the floor tonight—that way, I'll be able to feel something *hard* for a change!"

She smiled, nicely wriggled her way up from her computer, and asked, "Why do doctors slap babies' butts when they're born?"

"Um—why?"

"To knock the penises off of the smart ones!"

"But when you were born," I said, "The doctors likely took one look at you and slapped your parents instead."

I smiled. Karen giggled. She enticingly led the way back to the bedroom; and enticed, I followed the scenery. On the way in, I flicked on the stereo. Music helps me to relax during the time for loving. However, I lately do avoid these songs: *Banging on My Heart, Heart in Danger*, and especially *Hanging on a Heart Attack.*

Other than that, and despite the absence of our erotic toys, our bedroom ambiance is about the same. Oh—one more change: I replaced the *70 MPH* road sign that had hung over our bed with a *CAUTION* sign.

Luxuriously lying under that sign, Karen murmured, “Come here, you cancer slayer, you, you—Hun of my heart.”

I believe I lightly growled as I moved her way—growled and wished we had kept at least the “Naughty Nurse Outfit.”

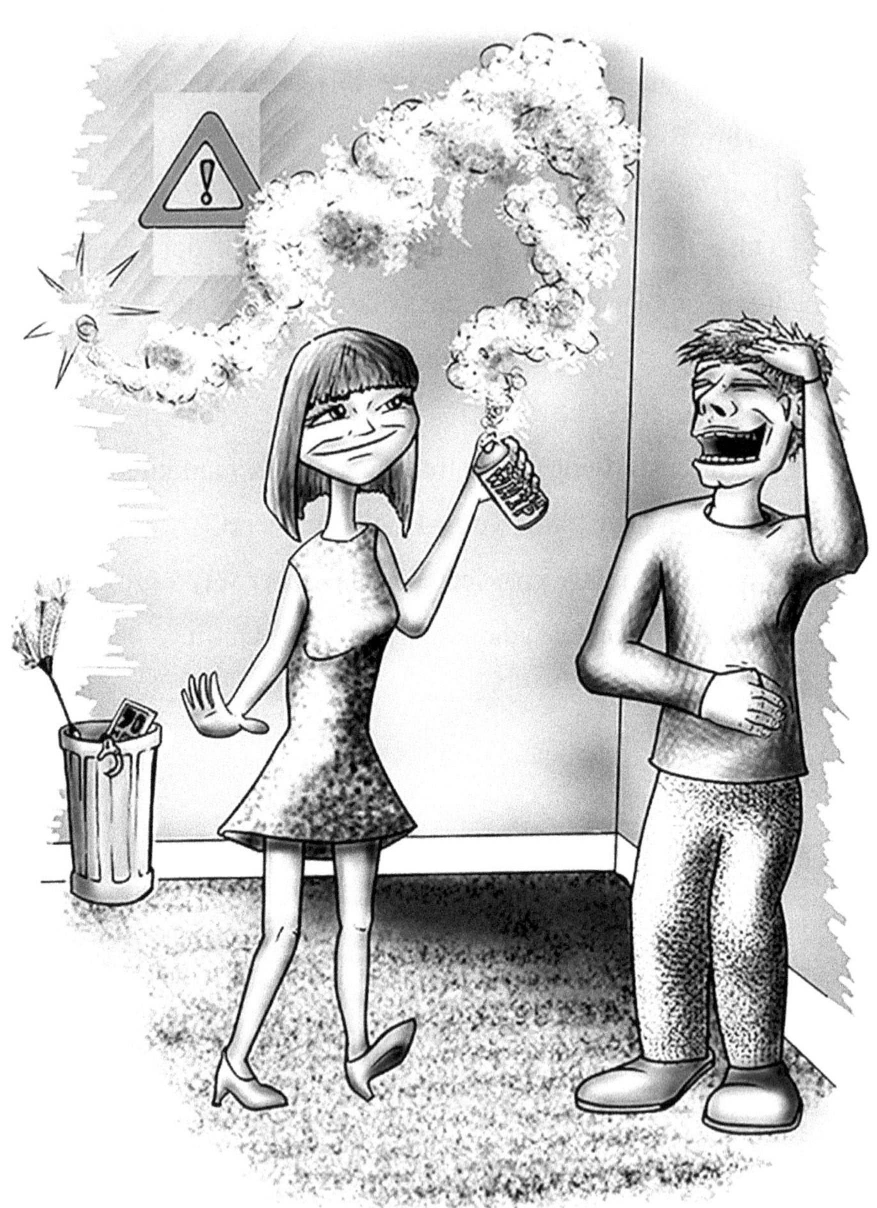

CHAPTER EIGHT

I'D *STILL* RATHER HAVE CANCER

To the living we owe respect, but to the dead we owe only the truth.
~ Voltaire

As we have seen, congestive heart failure is not *all* bad. It presents great incentives to avoid stress and to live healthily; and it allows for a moderated, yet maintainable love life.

It also expands the mental-list of songs that relate to *you*, the heart-conscious music connoisseur. Suddenly, I found myself listening intently when the radio or music channel played hearty songs that I had not before appreciated: Billy Ray Cyrus' A*chy Breaky Heart;* Stone Temple Pilots' *Trippin' on a Hole in a Paper Heart;* Nirvana's *Heart Shaped Box*; The Guess Who's *Heartbroken Bopper*; My Chemical Romance's *Bulletproof Heart*.

Hundreds of recorded songs have "heart" in the title, more of those hearts "achy-breaky" than bulletproof. It struck me that having heart problems had one big thing, with being in love. . . suddenly, *many* songs relate to *you,* the heart patient/the lover.

I am sure there are *also* songs about cancer. It is just that, other than Nirvana's "I wish that I could eat your cancer" line in *Heart Shaped Box*, I have not heard or noticed any. A cancer song seems right for a punkish or thrash-metal band ("You're like cancer, *gaaaaar-ar*") or maybe a rapper could repeatedly rhyme "cancer" with "dancer" and kind-of rhyme it with "danger" to create a rappin' danger dancer ho with killer cancer?

Musical variety aside, I'd still rather have cancer. Having, meaning *battling*, CANCER is like being a glory-sodden gladiator fighting to the death amidst the excited roar of the hero-worshipping crowd. By comparison, having CHF is like feverishly wasting away far beneath the arena in a cold, dark, damp, silent dungeon, unknown and unnoticed.

It does not arouse any interest, much less sympathy. The other day, outside of a grocery store, I saw a distant relative who had sent me a thoughtful card with $20 in it while I had been on chemo—a common kind of occurrence in those days. This time, he asked me if I would front him the funds for a twelve-pack, which I did.

"Thanks, cuz!" he beamed, and then he asked, "How have you been, anyway? I heard you beat your cancer but, jeez, you don't look so hot."

"Oh, it was cool beating cancer," I proudly said; "but the chemo that helped me beat it also damaged my heart, giving me congestive heart failure. I am trying to deal with that now, modifying my lifestyle."

"Oh yea? Whattaya know about that? Man, the other day I got into some poison oak—what a hassle! Look, I gotta run, but nice seeing you! Pay back that twenty anytime—but as soon as possible, okay cuz?"

Watching him hurry off, I thought about how he used to seem substantially older than I; now he seemed about the same age, which we are.

CHF is not the fund-raising boon like is cancer. I recently read of a lady in Chillicothe Ohio who had raised over $20,000 through a website and fundraisers to help with her cancer. The reason it made the newspaper is the reason she will need those funds is for a lawyer—*she never even had cancer*! Crafty crook, that lady. If she had tried the same scam with CHF, she would be in *bankruptcy*, not criminal court.

Another reason I'd rather have cancer is that you can chart and report your progress—if you are lucky enough to progress, which I was; if cancer had eaten my face off or killed me, I would of course have felt differently. The CT and PET scans had disclosed fewer and fewer outposts of cancer-cell desperados, until there were none. . . and oh, did I not shout *that* from the rooftops! Yes, I did . . .

until someone called the cops, that is; but the off-i-sher had slipped me a fiver *and* high-fived me!

I announced it all on Facebook, gaining hundreds of "likes" and dozens of congratulatory comments about "answered prayers," even from some known atheists.

How would I report "progress" on CHF? *Had fluid in my lungs this morning, but now its cleared. No sign of a heart attack yet.* Boring!

So, with cancer you can chart and report both progress and regress; but either way, you and your Facebook friends would see it coming from way off, by which time you would be the most popular Facebooker ever!

Not with heart failure—either it still beats, or it does not beat and—*bam!*—you are *gone baby gone*; and your Facebook friends, all ~~8~~, ~~7~~, 6 of them, could only wonder *why isn't what's-his-name on Facebook anymore?*

Cancer itself may not be fair—definitely is unfair—but at least it gives you relatively fair warning that it is coming to get you. A heart attack would drop from the sky like a bomb in a sneak attack. I know. In grad school we were told by a confused professor that calling Pearl Harbor a "sneak" attack is now considered politically incorrect because implying that the Japs were "sneaky" is somehow racist or something; but what the hell. . . it *was* sneaky and they *were* sneaks! And a heart attack is sneaky too—all ~~6~~, ~~5,~~ ~~4,~~ 3 of my Facebook friends agree with that.

Furthermore, when you have a healthy heart, but also a little cancer, charting your progress as you go, seeing your friendly oncologist frequently, they sure do treat you well in the cancer clinic's waiting room. Checking in, they broadly smile and ask if you would like a parking voucher. While you wait on comfy chairs among the other cancer superstars, some volunteer nearby gently strums a guitar or caresses the piano keys. The huge, tranquil aquarium in the corner holds beautifully exotic fish amidst its calming bubbles. The coffee vending machine, which *always* works, provides *free* gourmet coffee (or tea or hot chocolate). Thoughtfully placed wicker baskets are always filled with complimentary health-snacks and bottled water.

While waiting in this oh-so-soothing environment, you can browse through the in-house CARE catalog of their "survivorship" programs. This catalog has descriptions of *free* programs awaiting you, the Cancer VIP: everything from gardening to career counseling, acupuncture to reflexology to sexuality, yoga to meditation to music therapy.

It is nothing like that in the cardiology office. In the waiting room, sitting on hard chairs among scowling nobodies like yourself, you hear no soothing music, you see no tranquilizing fish-tank. You find no complimentary coffee or water or snacks, and they do not "greet" you so much as they "process" you.

For example, I recently checked in for my semi-monthly cardiologist appointment. The lady checking me in glanced up and said, "Oh—you again," and gazed back at her screen. She must have scanned my medical history because, a moment later, she muttered, "A *smoker*?"

I proudly thumped my chest and corrected her: "A *former* smoker!"

Not to be denied her dismal moment, she scowled and said, "Cancer cures smoking," before dismissively waving me off toward a hard-back chair.

Instead, I stood there and pulled out an electronic cigarette—I quit smoking, not vaporing. Blowing tobacco-flavored vapor at her, I said, "Cancel that appointment. *I'd rather have cancer* than to spend one more minute in this depressing place."

And I set off to find a cardiology clinic that would treat me like a cancer patient—that is, like a legendary celebrity. . .

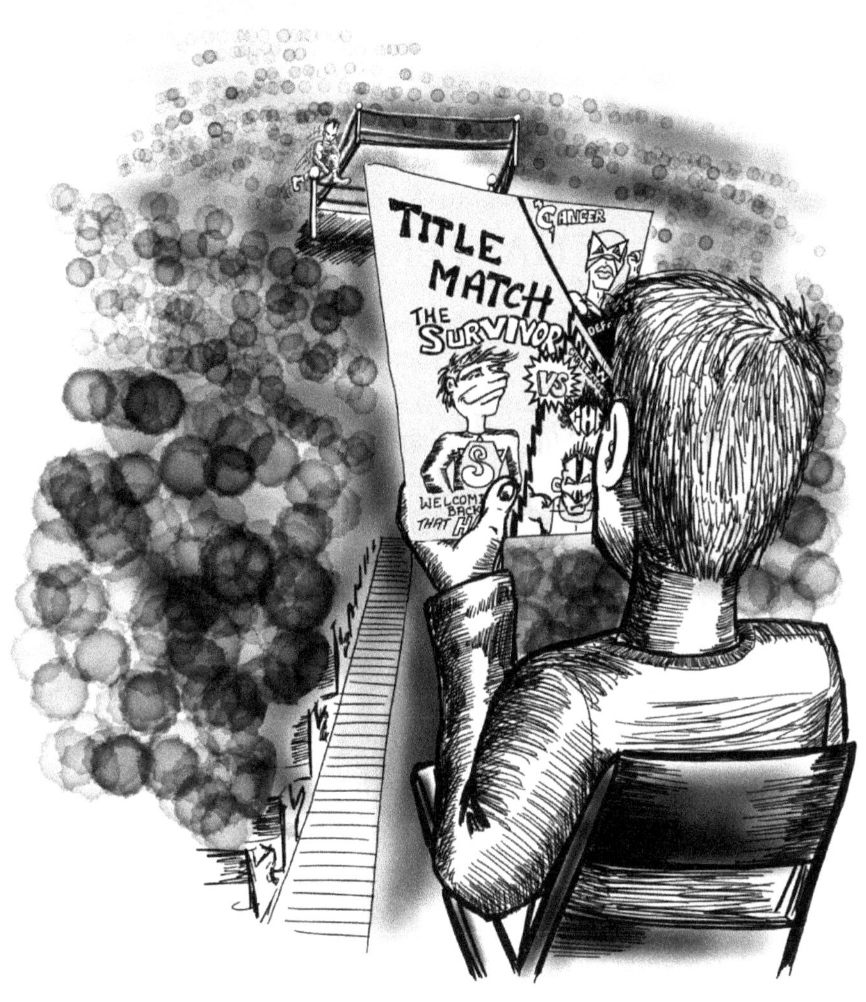
TITLE
MATCH
THE
SURVIVOR
VS
CANCER

CHAPTER NINE

STAND UP, OR SIT DOWN

The best doctors are Dr. Quietman, Dr. Dietman, and Dr. Merryman.
~ Jonathan Swift

So I needed a new cardiology clinic, and I *wanted* a cheerful one. Browsing the online yellow pages, I searched for a local one using search terms like "good humor." I recognized the name of one of the listed cardiologists, Dr. Jon Hart—I had seen him perform one Saturday night at the "Cork-N-Comics" club. If I remembered right, he seemed to have a twin onstage with him. No—no, in hindsight, that must have been me seeing double.

I called for an appointment, getting one for the next day with one of his partners. I do not know if this partner also did weekend stand-up but, sleepily arriving early for my first appointment, as Celine Dion crooned "My heart will go on" through overhead speakers, I quickly discovered that a comic mood reigned in the waiting room. Good: like with the cancer crowd, humor is needed in medical offices throughout sickdom. *Reader's Digest* claims monthly that "Laughter is the best medicine." Who are we to doubt them?

As I walked up to the brightly finger-painted receptionist's desk that seemed suitable for a daycare teacher, I eyed a wall poster hanging on the wall behind the desk:

WHEN YOU BREATHE, YOU INSPIRE
WHEN YOU DO NOT BREATHE, YOU EXPIRE

Suppressing a grin, I gave the cheery nurse/receptionist my name. She stared at the information on her screen and asked me how I had been feeling. Getting into the spirit of the place, I jested, "Except for my heart stopping now and then, I feel great!"

She smiled appreciatively. Celine Dion's song ended. . . and began again. . .

At the bordering registration desk, the receptionist handed a checking-out, overweight patient a bottle of orange pills, advising, "Do not consume these. Spill them on the floor three times a day and then pick them up one by one."

Good advice! My receptionist finished checking me in, started to hand me a dum-dum sucker, realized her mistake, and instead handed me a pamphlet (which I never did read). As "My Heart Will

Go On" ended again, and then started again, I found a padded chair and settled comfortably into it.

Nearby, two sixtyish women chatted. The one nearest me said, "I don't particularly care one way or the other, but where *is* your husband?"

The other lady whispered, "I thought you knew—he's *dead*!"

"Oh, I'll bet that he's just using that as an excuse!"

The widow thought for a moment and then replied, "I had such a time settling his estate—sometimes I wish he hadn't died at all!"

"My Heart Will Go On" ended again and—surprise!—began again. I rose to mention this to the receptionist.

When I arrived there, I had to wait, as a nervous-looking skinny man told her, "I'm very worried. I read last week that a man had entered the hospital over heart trouble but died there because of malaria!"

"Relax," she advised, gently patting his pencil-like arm and then pinching his pallid cheek. "*Our* clinic's hospital is top-notch. When you come in with heart trouble, *that's* how you'll die."

Finally, it was my turn. As "My Heart Will Go On" went on and on, I yanked myself out of a reverie and said, "With all respect, I think your music system has a defect. Ever since I arrived, it plays that song over and over again."

"Oh? The defect must be in *you*, sir. Our patients find that song uplifting, full of hope."

She then started humming to the music, even wriggling her elderly butt in her chair. She shut her eyes and swayed.

"Don't you think that maybe 'heart' is just a metaphor for emotional strength in those lyrics?" I asked.

She stopped humming and swaying, and she reopened her eyes.

"What are you? A music critic?"

I threw up my arms and walked away, and as I did, I thought I heard her mumble, "Because you're sure no writer."

My chair had been hijacked by an imp too young to have heart trouble, so I found another directly beneath this wall-sign:

IF YOUR TIME AIN'T COME,
NOT EVEN A DOCTOR CAN KILL YOU

I sat down. "My Heart Will Go On" ended. Silence momentarily followed, and then came the opening strains of Neil Young's "Heart of Gold."

A nurse appeared out of a door to my left and greeted a lightly coughing stooped guy who had an excellent handlebar mustache.

"Good afternoon, Mr. Burr," she said. "You seem to be coughing much more easily today."

Burr coughed, tweaked the tips of his mustache, and replied, "That's likely, because I spent all night practicing it."

"Heart of Gold" soulfully ended and Don Henley's "Heart of the Matter" soulfully began. Thinking that this place seemed a bit loony for a heart clinic, but also that I liked it for that reason, I went to examine their aquarium against a far wall. As I have mentioned, I had relished the restful effects of the cancer clinic's aquarium; and I was glad to see that the heart clinic included one too—this added some needed normalcy to its general lunacy. Getting closer, though, I noticed it was filled not with bubbly water but with dirty dirt! A plaque on it explained that this tank contained "inspirational" earthworms; apparently the worms "inspire" because, as the plaque explained, they have multiple hearts spread throughout their length, five in the average worm. Since I have ripped many worms in half to make my fishing bait last longer, I felt momentarily thankful that each piece likely had its own heart; this made me feel if not inspired, then at least less barbaric.

The bouncy opening strains of Rod Stewart's "This Old Heart of Mine" came on overhead—I sashayed some as I returned to my seat. Sitting there, for the second or third time since my arrival, I had a sudden sense of *Déjà vu.* In case this was some sort of sign of pending heart trouble, I started to rise to go tell the nurse-like receptionist; but seeing that she was right then enjoying a laugh with the other receptionist, I sat back down.

As the mysterious *Déjà vu* sensation wavered, half leaving and half lingering, an elderly all-grey gent accompanied by a white-smocked doctor exited one of the examination room doors.

The doc slapped the gent gently on his bent shoulder and said, "You're in *great* shape! I'd bet good money you'll live to be 80."

The gent blinked and said, "But Doctor Hart—I'm 80 right *now*!"

"See," the doc beamed, "What'd I tell you?"

I walked right by them on my way to the restroom as a new song came on: Motley Crue's "Doctor Feelgood." Inside the immaculately clean restroom were several small signs, including this one on the door:

FOR ASPHYXIATION:
APPLY ARTIFICIAL RESPIRATION UNTIL DEAD

I returned to the waiting room and, sure enough, someone had taken my chair. Indeed, looking around I noticed that nobody was sitting where they had originally sat, like in musical chairs. I also noticed that nearly all were smiling, or grinning, or at least smirking. I spotted an empty chair and moved that way. The receptionist, meanwhile, must have had her speakerphone on, because the whole room could now hear—over the bouncy tune of Roxette's "Listen to Your Heart"—a desperate-sounding man literally begging for an "emergency surgery" appointment.

Shaking her head so fiercely that her nurse's cap fell off, the receptionist informed him that no surgery was possible until a week from the next day.

You could hear the anxiety in the poor dude's amplified voice: "But—but—I might *die* before then!"

"No problem," the now-hatted nurse said, nodding and smiling, "If that happens, just call before to cancel the appointment."

I believe I heard inappropriate laughter as I settled into a chair that was empty except for an old copy of *MAD* magazine. I uneasily browsed through it, flipping pages to the throaty sounds of Bonnie Tyler's "Total Eclipse of the Heart."

After a time, Doctor Hart again escorted a patient, this one a handsome and sharply dressed man of about 30, all the way to the exit door, stopping just short of it.

"Go home and get a good night's sleep," Doctor Hart cheerily advised.

"Oh, sleeping's *not* the problem. It's when I get up—I feel dizzy for a half hour, and then I feel fine."

Doctor Hart momentarily pondered this, and then he said, "Well then, why don't you wait a half hour before getting up?"

The patient seemed to mull this over before saying, "I'd like a second opinion about *that*."

"Sure!" the doctor replied. "Come back tomorrow, and I'll give you another one!"

Then, as the guy turned to depart, the doc patted him on the rump. I deduced that Doctor Hart must be gay in *both* senses of the word.

As Celine Dion sang once again that her heart would go on, I started to wonder whether I truly wanted to be a patient of this crazy place. Still, I *had* enjoyed the attempted humor that floated so merrily around—humor had been one thing that I had liked about having cancer!

My eyes grew heavy.

I must have dozed off in the comfy chair. Opening my eyes, I observed that only I remained in the waiting room, other than the receptionist who stood directly above me, peering down.

"I'm sorry, young sir," she said (I love it when people call me 'sir'). "It seems we ran out of time before getting to you."

Rising from my chair, remembering all that I had witnessed here, I said," Hey, what kind of a heart clinic is this, anyway?"

"*Heart* clinic?" she chuckled. "Oh no, young man—this is 'Dr. Hart's *Comedy* Clinic'! I'm afraid you've been at the wrong place, albeit at the right time."

Oh—*that* explained it! "Well, it didn't seem all too *real*," I admitted.

"Yes," she said, prodding me toward the exit door. "It's time for you to get back to reality."

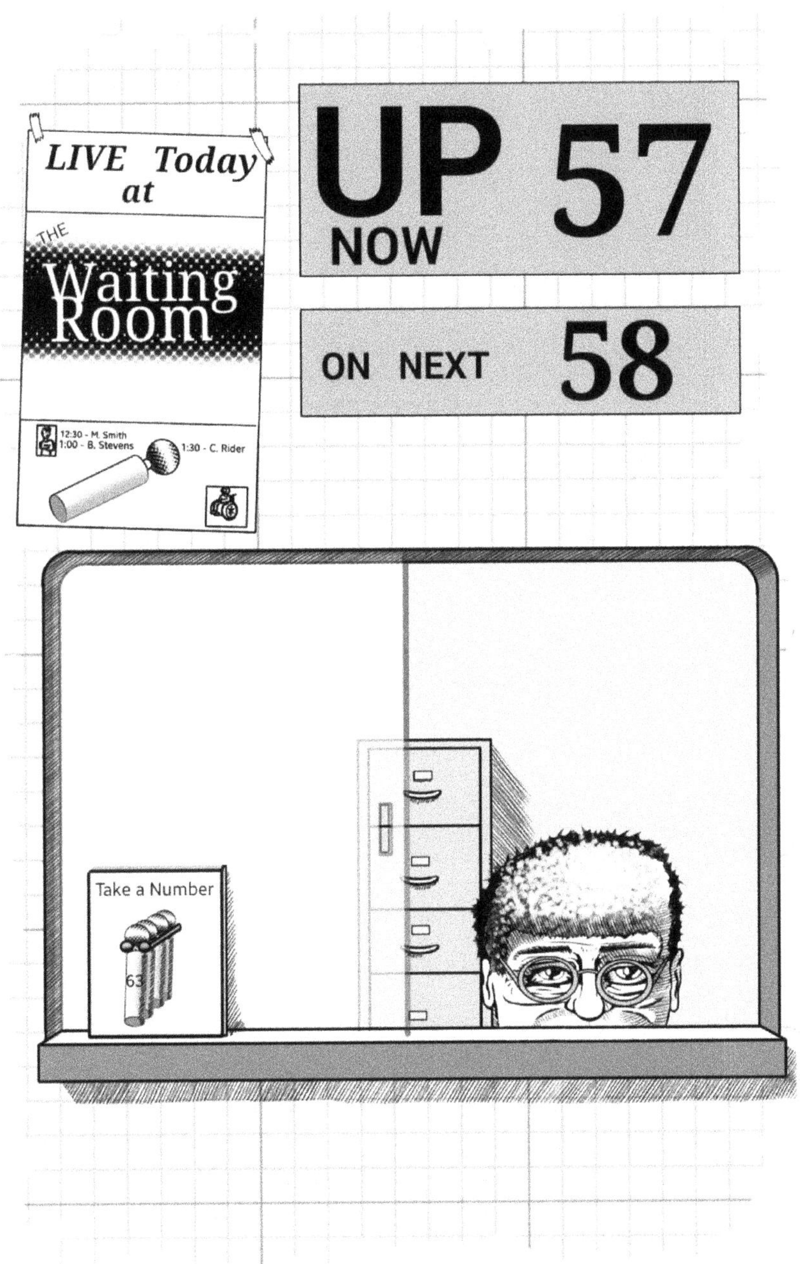
LIVE Today
at
THE
Waiting
Room
12:30 - M. Smith
1:00 - B. Stevens
1:30 - C. Rider
UP 57
NOW
ON NEXT 58
Take a Number
63

CHAPTER TEN

TWO GLASSES OF WHAT SIZE?

You never know what is enough unless you know what is more than enough. ~ William Blake

I sat back to my approximation of reality at home and started thinking about the birds and the bees—especially the bees. Do you know why bees congregate so busily around fallen rotting fruit such as pears? If you watched those bees very closely, you might notice a wobble to them. You see, bees and many other critters—including pigs, those involuntary donors of healthy heart valves—congregate gleefully about rotting fruit because such fruits are *fermenting*, creating alcohol.

Alcohol is natural, has a natural attraction to living creatures; and I naturally have always felt attracted to it, too. Oops—am I lunging away from reality again?

With my congestive heart challenge, the alcohol challenge is this: *moderation.* Moderation had always seemed like good advice that I sometimes tried to take; and now it was a *requirement* should I care to live beyond, say, next weekend.

I too have heard the rumors—undoubtedly spread by the vineyards' associations—that two glasses of red wine might even be *good* for one's heart health, so I had sought for facts to back up the promising rumor.

I found them, too. It seems that grape-skins (which are used in making red—not white—wine) contain an anti-oxidant called "resveratrol" that has several heart-helping properties. Of course, simply eating red grapes will supply you with resveratrol, too.

However, then you would forego the other, substantial heart benefits of *any* form of alcohol: raises levels of "good" cholesterol, reduces the formation of blood clots, decreases inflammation, relaxes you, prompts you to perform aerobic exertion while impressing that appealing babe with your dazzling dance moves—oh, wait, we are still talking about *moderate* amounts of booze here, like two glasses. Regarding babes, *one* glass is recommended for women. It seems that men have more of an alcohol-metabolizing enzyme. That is why most men can drink most women under the table, perhaps hoping for a kiss while we're down there.

Not everyone agrees that glasses of alcohol are good for you. For instance, the *American Heart* Association, which never gave me even a dime, asserts that there is no scientific proof that *any* amount of alcohol can replace more conventional (aka *boring*) measures toward heart health.The spoil-sports! On the other hand, the cancer societies are much more liberal, not making such a big deal about their cancer warriors enjoying a drink or two.

When I was on a chemo-schedule, I would get chemo on Thursdays and start taking prescribed nausea-reducing, energy-boosting steroids on Fridays. That set up Saturdays, autumn Saturdays in my case. Hyped on steroids, afternoons I would work-out watching college football, barbarically screaming at the screen on occasion, and then drink beer watching more college football at night. Don't even ask about *Sundays* during my chemo period!

That is another way, I thought, that CHF makes me feel older than I ever did with cancer—all I have now are memories, when my whole life I have preferred *making* memories.

I poured my first glass of red wine. Not many stories in *that*, so while I sipped I thought of some stories past . . .

I never drank like I drank when I attended, usually, the Ohio State University as an over-aged undergraduate. The twenty-year-old students at the campus apartment complex had quickly appraised me as someone nearly as old as their parents, but way cooler. They also seemed to value me as someone who did not even need an ID to legally obtain beer and other adult beverages for their drinking pleasures.

I soon found myself meeting more smiling 20-year-olds than I ever knew existed. I took many rides to local beer docks where I obtained massive amounts of beer for them, and a moderate amount of always complimentary brew for me. I was invited to, and even sometimes starred at numerous bashes.

By the end of that first semester, I was barely hanging on to my health, my sanity, and my stellar academic standing. I decided to move back with my parents who were, believe it or not, even older than I, and way milder than the 20-year-old buckeyes.

The semester ended one week before the end of the year. I could not go out so timidly and quietly!

Having just received my financial aid for the *next* semester, when I would not need much money except for a little to repay bounced checks, I looked over at my roomie, Russell Bryan, dazedly lounging on our stained couch that reeked of stale beer—we had tried to burn it after the Michigan game; but it had refused to catch fire—and I said, "Want to drive me to get a keg?"

Russell was a moderately tall, stylishly thin, thoroughly good-looking dude. He had arrived as a freshman on full scholarship because of his near-perfect ACT score (because he was a very intelligent dude) but now he loitered on academic probation (because he was also a very wild man).

In answer to my question, he raised one eyebrow and then the other one. Next I heard jangling keys. Before long, we were back on our own turf, just we two, a keg of beer, and a large mushroom pizza. I turned down the stereo sounds—Alice in Chains—as Russell put his cell phone to use and summarized, over and over, our cozy little scenario, which became a *crowded* scenario before too long.

At least 50 or 60 vacationing students had flocked back to campus, and we all had a terrific time. The next morning was the day before New Year's Eve. Being out of coffee, Russell and I and a half-dozen stay-overs polished off the remains of the keg and went merrily for two more. That day *and* night, we did not need to call anyone—they just showed up, maybe 150 vacationing students festively filling our apartment and the two neighboring ones.

The day after *that*, I felt like it might be time to quit; but only I did, plus this was *not* the time to quit, it being the promising morning of New Year's Eve. The guys laughed when I ordered a six-pack with the three kegs—for the ride back. And it was a good thing that we got *three* kegs this time, because someone stole one at some point during the crazed night.

Only two or three fights broke out, but these did not last long. At one point, I edged into a big circle of boisterous partiers, mostly guys, surrounding and cheering on something, I figured another fight. When I reached the inner circle, I found the cause of the excitement—two girls embracing and kissing.

We were all still going strong when the New Year arrived, some of us singing Prince's "Tonight I'm gonna party like it's

1999"—because it *was* 1999! I do not remember *anything* after that, other than that the partying went on and intoxicatingly on …

The next morning—mid-afternoon, actually—things were not nearly as festive, but they were *okay* when Russell produced a pint he had saved for such an occasion. He and I and several other dudes sipped it and sighed.

Then Russell's blue eyes lit, and I figured he must be recalling a scene from the previous night. He glanced my way, sipped, and passed me the pint.

"Man oh man," he said, lightly punching my shoulder. "I never would have guessed that my roomie likes to party *naked*!"

At the moment, fully clothed, I took another sip of wine and smiled at that then-embarrassing, now-satisfying recollection.

I have had great eras of drinking other than at Ohio State. One such era had been when I first started writing a lot and publishing a little, when it seemed that even the sky was 'no limit.' During this era, I hanged and drank with a German-American named Juan.

Founder and sole surviving member of the short-lived organization DAMM (*Drunks against Mad Mothers*) Juan would surely help me with recollections of drinking stories. I had not talked with him for a few years, so he probably had some new ones. I took another sip—2/3 gone!—and gave him a call.

"Hey Juan, it's me, your idol!"

He sounded suitably inebriated.

"*You*? I thought that you were *dead* or something. Didn't you have, what was it, liver cancer, maybe?"

"No Juan, *my* liver is fine—how's yours? Do you still drink all the time?"

"All the time? *Hell* no—I have to sleep, too, right? Anyway, beer still is the reason I get up every afternoon. Why do you ask? You're starting to sound like my dad."

Juan is a professional cartoonist, meaning that he still lives with his parent. I smiled, thinking of Juan's righteous papa, not only a tee-totaler, but an anti-drinking one.

"How is your dad?" I asked. "Still thumping the bible at you?"

I heard a bottle being gulped, an abbreviated burp, and then this: "Well, not so much lately. A couple weeks ago he had been watching this History channel program on Jesus' life and times. Afterwards he barged into my room and announced, 'I'm not so sure about Jesus anymore.'"

"Oh, no! Why?"

"That's what I'm getting at, pod. I asked him that; and he said, sadly shaking his head, 'I cannot believe it—changing water into *alcohol*.' He's been in a daze ever since, some sort of spiritual crisis, I suppose. Enough about him—what's up with you?"

"Not much. I thought you'd help me remember some old drinking scenes."

You see, Juan and I used to drink at what we called "Twelve-pack hot spots." It started with our realization that some places—riverbanks and rooftops—are downright *cool* for drinking beer. Once we had the basic concept, though, we had escalated it, drinking beer at places such as the top of the local water tower and the flat-top roof of the local jail.

But Juan was not in the story-telling mood.

Instead, he said, "So, you beat your cancer's butt, huh? Cheers! I'll bet you drink to that victory, huh? Now that you're out of danger, it's—what?—bottoms up?"

"Um, well, Juan," I began, "actually, I drank a respectable amount while stomping cancer, but chemo left me with a *heart* issue; so I'm cutting way back on booze."

"*Booze*—did you say *booze*? I love the sound of that! Loosey-goosey, boozie-woozie! So, pod, cancer, heart issue, what's the diff?"

"Well, actually a pretty big one. I—"

"There is no *real* diff," he interrupted. "Don't start living like you're already dead, bro. Live like you did before cancer and with cancer. . . keep on living like you're dying!"

"Aw, Juan, I haven't given up or anything. Hell, I'm drinking some vino right this minute!"

"What—two glasses, right?"

"Yep!"

"But—two glasses of what size?" he said, chuckling. He then added, "Hey, Big Ben—you remember him, right?—is coming by here soon. How bout we meet you at a bar halfway between here and there—or at that new pizza-pub near you? I'll buy you the biggest glass of wine they have!"

"Uh, no," I replied. "Every time I go to someplace like that, everybody wants to buy me drinks to toast to my having beaten cancer."

"What the hell is wrong with that?"

"Well—"

"Okay, I'll tell you what. Me and Big Ben will come over there. I have a gift for you, anyway."

"Let me guess—a bottle or a twelve-pack?"

"Oh no, pod. We'll see you in about a half hour."

An *hour* and a half later, a tremendous pounding rattled my back door. I let the barbarous door-pounders inside: Juan, a muscle-bound bruiser with military-cut blonde hair and a permanent sneer, and Big Ben, built like Juan but on a taller frame, with a recent beard, perhaps to make up for the hair no longer on the top of his head. Juan carried a gift-wrapped box, and Big Ben carried a twelve-pack in one meaty hand, two bottles of probable wine in the other hand.

"What took you guys so long?"

"Oh—we had to walk," said Juan. "Benny-*boy* here refused to be my DDD for the night."

"DDD?"

"Designated *drunk* driver" Benny said, grinning as he headed toward the fridge. "But I gave that up—it was too wasteful spilling my drinks every bump!"

He soon returned with two beers and one of the bottles of probable wine, which he placed in front of me. "It's my own from last year. Black raspberry—it has a touch of redness to it!"

He nodded his big head as if in approval.

"Sure does," I said, eyeing it.

Pointing at the "Happy Birthday" themed gift-wrapped package, I then asked Juan what it might be.

"Open it and see!" he directed.

So, I removed that tissue wrapping, opened the rectangular box within, and extracted the two largest wine glasses I have ever seen.

"They hold a fifth apiece," Juan proudly said. "Guess *that* solves your little conundrum with only two glasses a night."

Next he filled one by emptying the nearby fifth of wine into it.

Juan pulled out a cigarette, a "100" by the look of it.

"I'm sure you don't smoke anymore," he said, reaching in his pocket for a lighter. "They say one smoke takes five minutes off your life. But *these*," he continued, holding up the long cigarette, "take ten minutes to smoke, so I figure I'm five minutes ahead on each one. Mind if I light up in here?"

"I don't think so, Juan," Benny said. "It smells too much like cinnamon in here for a smoking room."

I did not say anything to that—lately, I had been puffing cinnamon-flavored e-cigs.

"Let's go out to the patio," I instead suggested, as I lifted the huge wineglass. "I want to show you my plants anyway."

"Oh well," Juan said, rising. "I'm getting used to the idea that by the time I go there, hell will be the only place left where smoking is allowed!"

"That's why I suggest that you go there all the time," remarked Benny, patting Juan's back as he followed us out to the plant-lined deck. "So, that you'll be someplace where you feel comfortable."

"Speaking of *comfortable. . .* " Juan said, gazing about the torch- lit deck, at the gorgeous potted tomato and pepper plants and the padded chairs of the patio set that Karen had bought for my birthday.

Once settled into those comfy chairs, we laughed a lot and recollected stories of crazed times past. I just cannot now remember what any of them were, other than that several involved the kicking in of doors, one kicked-in door leading to jail (Juan) and another to the emergency room for a fractured ankle (me). I *am* certain I did not "party naked" this time. (I do *that* only with Karen now, and those scenes are mercifully censored.)

Eventually, the boys decided that it was too late, and they were too inebriated, to trudge or wobble home. Big Ben claimed the couch while Juan chose the carpeted floor, mumbling that this would be one bed he could not fall off.

In the bedroom, falling into sleep, I felt fleeting uneasiness; because sprawled dudes and emptied bottles might trip-up Karen's early morning arrival. However, the uneasiness soon faded, in coordination with my own contented fading away.

In vino veritas? When drinking wine, the quantity in the glass is not nearly as important as the quality of the company with whom one drinks.

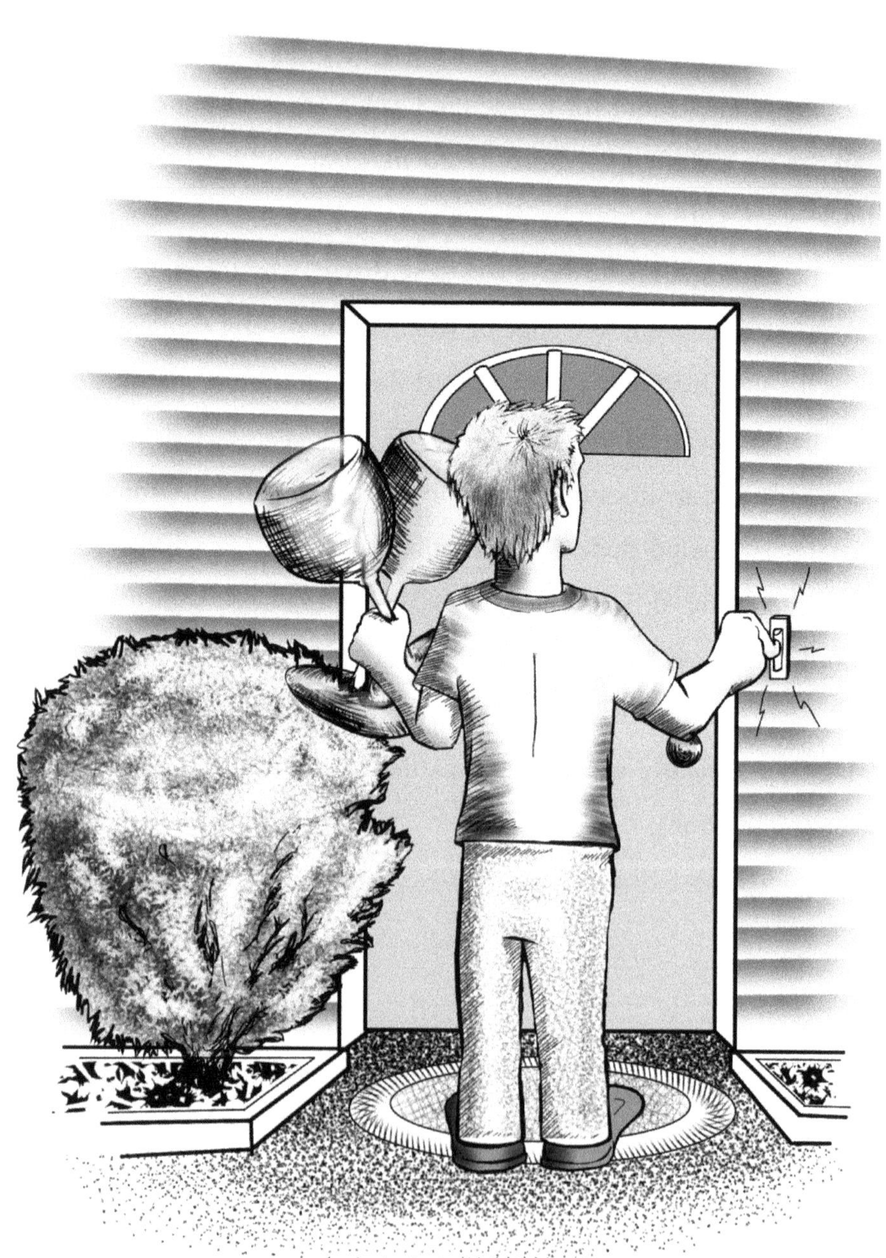

CHAPTER ELEVEN

APPETIZERS

The West wasn't won on salad.
~ North Dakota Beef Council ad

When Karen arrived the next morning, we were still sprawled out, all over the place although Big Ben no longer was sprawled on the couch—he had, at some point, found a bed, it being my *flower* bed out front. He sheepishly followed Karen in, he grinning and she grimacing; both of them had a flower in their hair, his accidental but hers intentional.

Juan arose from the couch quickly with Karen poised over him holding a tilted glass of ice water. She looked lovely in a flowered summer dress and that freshly-cut flower in her freshly brushed auburn hair that looked extra fresh next to Juan with his sleep-crazed hair.

Perhaps seeking to impress her, yet clearly not knowing how, he instantly started boasting about the supposedly titanic quantities of alcohol we had consumed the night before. Not only did that *not* impress her, but she had to already know, with mostly-empty beer and wine bottles all about—on the coffee table, the end tables, the bookshelves.

Still, she smiled. She sweetly asked Juan how much *I* had drank.

Juan grinned, glanced at me, and said, "Aw, that lightweight? Just one, maybe two glasses of wine."

But Karen, who had by then toured the apartment, then asked, "One or two glasses of *what* size?"

The guys soon departed, eyes now gleaming with plans—I kind of wanted to accompany them. However, Karen and I had plans of our own. After discarding the empty bottles, I poured my second cup of coffee and sat down with her at our round wooden table, actually a sized-for-two "ice cream table" set with heart-shaped chair-backs.

Karen started right in: "It's not just alcohol you need to watch, *hon-ee*, with your heart condition; caffeine is something else you should cut back on. You'll live longer! I want to have you for a long, long time!"

"When I give up coffee and drinking and everything else, I would not *want* to live a 'long, long time,'" I countered, taking an ample sip, scorching my tongue and spritzing some onto the polished table.

Karen watched this demonstration of klutziness a moment, and then said, "Aren't *I*—*we*—reason enough to live longer?"

I answered, "Yes, especially if you and I are enjoying a coffee or a glass of wine together."

"And—what about if we *do* decide to have children? You would want to live long enough to watch them grow up—all of them with curly hair, blue eyes, and crooked noses, just like you!"

She leaned over and kissed my crooked nose.

The idea did appeal to me. Kids are okay, but babies are super-duper!

"So," I said, puffing up, "You think I'd make a good daddy, right?"

"Yea, sure," she said, grinning, "Especially if our baby liked to go out drinking!"

I smiled. She smiled. Eye to eye, I decided to *not* remind her we were too old to start a family. We kissed. Then we showered, finalized our grocery list, and headed out.

We had not "finalized" our list, after all. On the road to the store, Karen driving "because your alcohol-blood level is probably still above the limit," we modified that list, meaning we expanded it. Perhaps we should have eaten before leaving. For instance, Halloween was yet a long way off, but we added trick-or-treat type sweets to our list, but not for costumed kids—not unless Karen had sneakily purchased another "naughty nurse" outfit.

On my chemo-diet, I had always bought whatever appeared appetizing, eating nearly none of it. Most of my previously favorite foods had suddenly tasted like do-do. On chemo, if only junk food had tasted good to me—if only barbequed earthworms had tasted good—that is what I would eat. A few bites.

With my appetite now closer to normal, but with my heart pumping at sub-normal, I needed to emphasize low-sodium, high fiber, and high potassium—bananas, strawberries, tomatoes. Always inclined to eat healthily to begin with, I had no real problem with the new recommended diet, other than that health foods lack preservatives, and I now felt I could use some preserving!

These kinds of thoughts occupied me as I pushed the cart and followed Karen through the produce section. I adore the colors and shapes of produce sections! Alas, when I reached to squeeze one of the cantaloupes, it seems I squeezed Karen's rounded rear instead! (I really should *always* wear my contact lens.) She made a noise like a cantaloupe never has!

Karen had researched nutrition so extensively during my cancer and now with my CHF, that it had changed *her* diet. She was now a vegetarian. She does not eat anything that can have children.

Eyeing her as *she* eyed the bananas, I said, "Hey! I don't remember seeing *dog food* on the list!"

She gave me a sarcastic *ha-ha* as she selected a slightly greenish bunch. You see, it had not been enough for Karen, *herself,* to become a vegetarian; now her erstwhile cocker spaniel, Wagster, was involuntarily a vegetarian too! Although he did not choose this novel doggy diet, he stoically takes what he finds in his food bowl.

I had once been a vegetarian, naturally when I had lived in unnatural Southern California. I was *still* a vegetarian a few years later when I undertook my first cross-country bicycle tour—from the heart of Ohio to the coast of California. During a bicycle tour, as your legs build muscles upon muscles, you have an increased protein need; however, on such a tour you have a harder time managing the "protein compliments," such as combinations of rice and beans (grains and legumes) that vegetarians need to fit into their diet for adequate protein.

I had not even thought of eating a hamburger for years, but passing by a Burger King in Grants Pass, New Mexico, the aroma of flame-broiled flesh slowed and then stopped me. Shortly after that, I was propped under a desert tree in a small park across from Burger King devouring a *lovely* "Whopper"—my first burger in years. Then I had my second burger in years. Then, after a short nap I pedaled westward.

Now I do eat meat. Like with wine, sex, and exercise, I just do it in moderation. I still *prefer* fruits and veggies. Think of it this way: animals we might like to devour have ways to escape or repel us and our appetites—the rabbit's elusiveness, the pheasant's camouflage, the pig's ugliness; meanwhile fruits and veggies, with exotic, if not erotic shapes, *and* vivid colors lure us, seduce us, and seemingly *beg* us to sample them. Now, if only fruits and veggies had aromas as alluring as sizzling bacon!

Finally back in my apartment's soul kitchen, the groceries put away, the wine chilling, and Wagster staring quizzically at his food bowl in which I had placed some bananas and an orange, we set about double-teaming a batch of eggplant/zucchini parmesan. I started the bowl of sauce and spices while Karen, slap-happy with the wooden spatula, got the oil heating for frying the sliced eggplant and zucchini. "Hey," she said, smacking my rear with the spatula, "aren't fried foods *bad* for you?"

I smiled. "Karen, what kind of oil will you fry them in?"

"Um—olive oil."

"See? Olives are *vegetables*—it's gotta be good for you!"

Whap, whap!

She eventually had to use the whap-whapping spatula in that oil. Rather than describe the detailed preparations here, and so that you could sample the delectable results for yourself, here is our own semi-famous recipe for Layered Eggplant/Zucchini Parmesan …

LAYERED EGGPLANT/ZUCHINI PARMESAN

Ingredients:

- 2 med. eggplants; or 3 med. zucchini; or some combination of the two
- 8 ounces of sliced mushrooms
- 1 sweet bell pepper
- 1 med. sweet onion
- Flour
- Oil (olive oil preferred)
- Italian dressing
- 2 med. cans of tomato sauce
- 1 med. can of crushed tomatoes
- 1 small can of tomato paste
- Garlic (powder or crushed/minced—use plenty)
- Other Italian herbs/spices(basil, crushed peppers, etc.) to taste
- Parmesan cheese
- Mozzarella cheese
- Angel hair pasta

Step one: In large bowl, thoroughly mix the tomato products, the garlic, the Italian herbs/spices, and the parmesan cheese—plenty of that (1/2 to 2/3 cup). Also stir in several tablespoons of Italian dressing.

Step two: Sauté the sliced strips of bell pepper, sliced onion, and sliced mushrooms. When done, add to the sauce mix.

Step three:

1. Preheat oven to 350 degrees
2. Bread and lightly fry ¼" to ½" slices of eggplant and/or zucchini

Step four:

1. Place layer of sauce-mix at bottom of greased baking pan
2. As eggplant/zucchini gets done, place on bottom layer of sauce

3. After bottom layer filled with fried eggplant/zucchini, place another layer of sauce-mix on it, and then add an additional layer of eggplant/zucchini (probably two, possibly three layers to a pan)
4. Add layer of sauce-mix to the top of the last layer of eggplant/zucchini

Step five:

1. Cover pan with foil and bake 40 minutes
2. Cook angel-hair (or thin) pasta

Step six:

1. Remove pan from stove; remove foil from pan
2. Top with a layer of mozzarella cheese
3. Bake uncovered 5 to 10 additional minutes

Serving:

- ✓ Pasta on the side for excess sauce
- ✓ *Great* with
  - ➢ Garlic bread
  - ➢ Salad
  - ➢ Wine

If you tried—or will try—doing it alone, you will understand why we recommend double-teaming it. Speaking of that, with the dishes clean and put away, we double-teamed a bottle of *Stella Rosa* wine. Karen actually used one of my huge wine glasses as we relaxed to music. She also playfully used the now-clean wooden whapping spatula after I playfully jerked the girlish ponytail that she had tied for working in the kitchen.

It had been a splendid day and evening, but it was not over yet. What next? We polished off the wine and headed for the other room, the one with the **CAUTION** sign, where we worked off our meal, exercising no caution in the process.

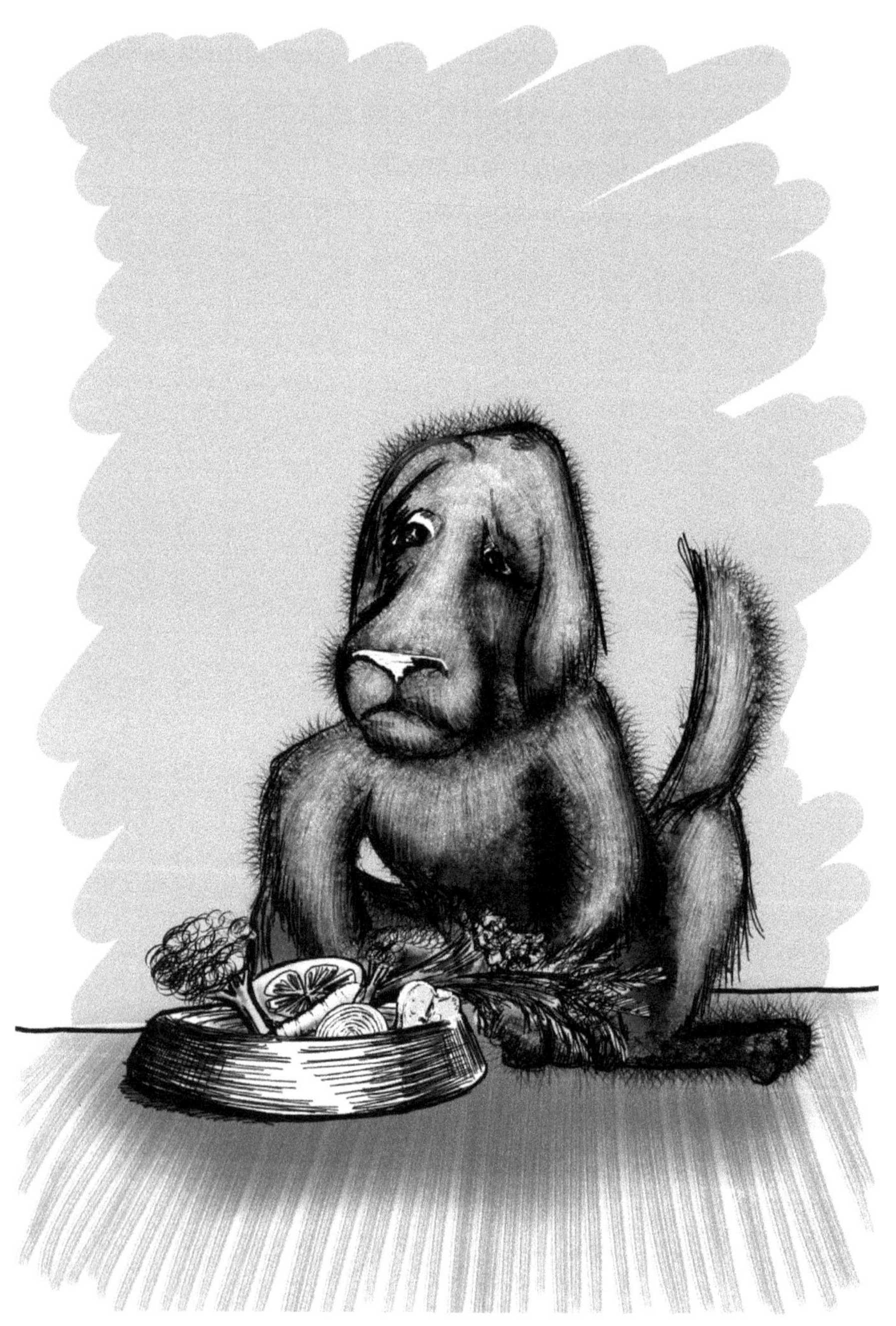

CHAPTER TWELVE

DUMBBELLS AND ME

Anything worth doing is worth doing slowly.
~ Mae West

Several mornings later, I noticed in the leering mirror that my mid-section had expanded to beyond-healthy proportions. I *had* looked skeletal toward the end of my chemo period and was pleased to be beyond that; however, I had bulged way beyond it to the point where Karen had teasingly taken to calling me "dumpling," and I could see why! Whereas chemo rendered me nauseous over good, wholesome food, CHF allows me to enjoy seconds and thirds of cuisine such as the aforementioned eggplant/zucchini parmesan, as well as anything and everything for dessert.

I had been walking up to several miles a day, but it seemed time to up the stakes, to start a moderate yet steady workout regime. I knew that Karen was, as usual, online; so I said from across the room, "Hey baby, look up 'congestive heart failure and exercise,' will you?"

"Okay!" she happily replied—Karen loves looking up information. Bring up *any* topic, and she will have the low-down on it in no time. If not for her, I would have missed National Eat-a-Pickle Day and would be ignorantly unaware of what is the Ohio State Insect (ladybug).

Several minutes later she blurted, "I found it! Listen to this, darling: 'Sex counts as exercise. It uses about five calories per minute. Plus. . . "

"*Whoa* baby! What did you use as search terms?"

"'Sex' and 'exercise' and 'heart:' isn't that what you wanted?"

"Well, not exactly," I answered, smiling at her.

"Plus, you just interrupted me! There's more here about sex and your heart. Did you know that sex lowers your blood pressure?"

"It lowers *something*," I admitted, peering over her tan shoulder, and then lightly kissing it. "What's this? The average man's heart is ten ounces and the average woman's eight ounces? I told you I have a bigger heart!"

"Hold on, buckaroo—I am *not* an 'average woman.' Plus, read on—sex helps women's bladder control. When a woman has an orgasm, it causes contractions in pelvic floor muscles, working them out, *strengthening* them. Don't think only of yourself, sweet-pea!"

She reached back and smacked my rear—still slaphappy, that's Karen, and she added, "Now that you've beaten cancer, you should think of *my* needs, too!"

What could I say to that?

"I *am* thinking of you, baby," I said, rubbing her shoulder as she purred. "As a matter of fact, I'm wondering how you'd like to go *shopping*."

Oh yea, I know what Karen likes—she literally leaped out of her chair. "What would I be shopping for?" she asked excitedly.

"Some weights, baby. Like a pair of dumbbells."

"How appropriate! Dumbbells of what size?"

"Let's see—about 25 pounds each, to start."

"Okay, two 25 pound dumbbells, Tarzan. Are those like long bars with weights at the end?"

"No baby, those are barbells. Dumbbells are the small short ones with the weights pre-attached."

"Oh," she nodded, starting to smile wide, dimples deepening. "I see—*dumbbells.* Like the ladies use?" Then she pinched my cheek and winked and asked, "Would you like to use one of my workout outfits while you're at it?"

"You mean one of your nighties or one of your shopping outfits? Sex and shopping are the main workouts that you get!"

"Yea—and I don't get enough of *either*," she said with a fake pout that she had gotten quite good at doing.

She then gathered her things and headed out the door, her rounded hips getting a workout as she went.

I turned on the stereo, poured another coffee, and sat down to Karen's computer. I used the *right* search terms this time and soon found out what the doctor had implied, and I could have guessed: with CHF, you should start a gradual, progressive training program—again, moderation in all things, including this. I eyed the giant wineglasses—maybe I could store my dumbbells in those?

I also read that the heart is nearly all muscle and is strong enough to lift 3,000 pounds, roughly the weight of a compact car. That would be an *undamaged* heart, I figured—my damaged one could likely lift about 50 pounds of dumbbells. I used to work out for an hour and then rest for ten. I suspected that would now be reversed, working out for ten minutes and then recuperating for an hour.

Just as I got prepared to do some toe-lifts, my phone rang. My caller ID identified Juan as the caller.

"Hey Juanito! What's the haps?"

"Bambino! I just woke up to some liquid lunch. Whatcha doin'?"

"Oh, reading up on what type of exercise is good for my wounded heart—it looks like aerobics might be good."

"Yep, aerobics will help you to convert fats, sugars, and starches into aches, pains, and cramps! What are you worried about, anyway? You've *always* been in pretty good shape."

"Aw, for months after my tumor-removal surgery I was forbidden to lift over five pounds. Then chemo weakened me, and now this heart failure bullshit makes me feel like I need to eat right, sleep right, and work out just to feel about as good as I used to feel with a mild hangover."

"Wah-wah-*wah*! Man, you used to party with me till two in the morning and then bicycle twenty miles to work four or five hours later."

"Yea, and now I go to cancer walk-a-thons. People may think I am doing it for cancer, but I do it for the exercise!"

"Lately, the only thing I've exercised is caution," Juan said. "But I did start a strict exercise regimen yesterday. So far I've missed only one day!"

"So far, so good, huh? What's this 'regimen' consist of Juan? Jumping to conclusions?"

"Oh, that and, um, carrying things too far."

I thought for a moment, and then I said, "What about dodging responsibilities? That's exercise!"

"Right on, bro. Plus, pushing my luck. *That's* a workout and a half!"

"Sure, but—no running?"

"Well, yea bro—running late! Why run, anyway? You'd only die tired."

"Yep, I've noticed some of my old high-school classmates who have jogged for years, hobbling about town looking dead tired."

"I know! I walked up on a crooked old guy the other day tap-tapping his cane. I was going to offer to help him to cross the street. Turns out it was Tim Tupelo, three years younger than me, winner of countless 5-Ks!"

"Sure," I agreed. "I'm going back to bicycling, *after* getting in shape with long walks. I started daily walks several months back and love it. It's a great idea-prompter, too."

"Ah, walking—I like it too. I think that's the main reason we have legs. Plus, I've never gotten stopped for walking while intoxicated. Well, once, but they didn't arrest me! You don't have to buy any equipment for walking, and it doesn't wear you out. Yet, most people wouldn't walk at all if not for walking their dogs. Speaking of walking, pod, it's time for me to walk on down to the corner store for a couple of 40-ounce weights to lift lip-ward this afternoon."

"See ya, bub." After flipping shut my phone, I again eyed the huge wineglasses. Filled up, how much might they weigh?

No, no. . . the time had arrived to start getting into shape, slowly but surely. The only thing was that indoors exercise had always seemed boring. I figured walking and cycling would be my main events, enjoying scenery as I went, perhaps coming up with some worthwhile ideas too. Indoors, I could do toe-lifts and pump or curl the dumbbells—in front of the TV (an idea I had while walking the other day). Baseball games, for example, take three hours, and so working out while watching the Tribe would make that less wasteful of time, especially when they lose, which does happen.

Since the Tribe had a night game this day, it felt like time for a walk—except for just then Karen breezed in carrying hot-pink dumbbells and saying, "I think I'll start pumping iron, too!"

From the look in Karen's eyes, my only walk right then would be to the bedroom—her idea of our exercise room, albeit not for pumping iron.

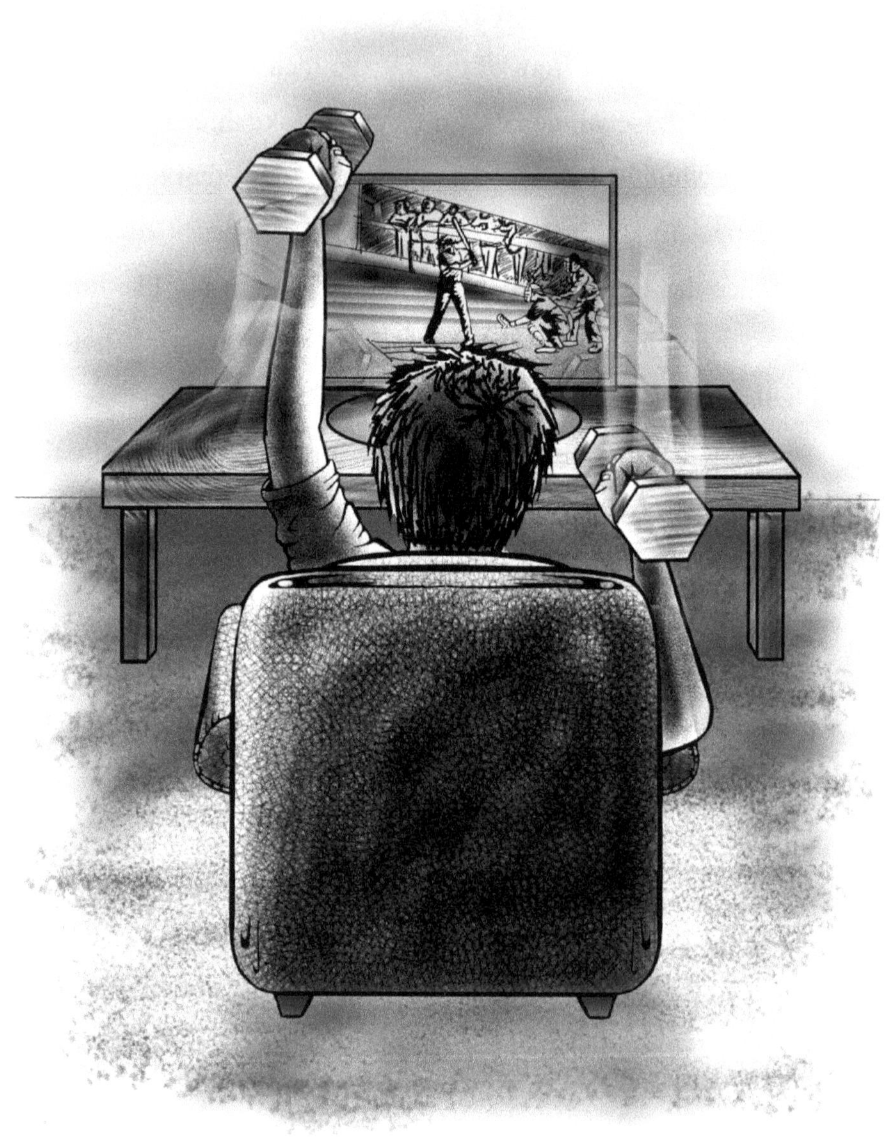

CHAPTER THIRTEEN

OH, THE THINGS I'LL DO

If the bell rings, why should we run?
~ Thoreau

"How do you spend your time lately?" my oncologist's nurse asked during my latest post-scan visit.

"Well, I'm writing another book," I said.

A moment of silence followed while she blankly stared at me, apparently waiting for more.

"Books don't grow on trees you know," I sternly added.

"Yes, I'm sure, but you can't write *all* day," she confidently asserted; and she then less confidently added, "Can you?"

"True," I said, and I left it at that, privately pondering the day-to-day activities that leisurely fill my days. . .

I do walk a lot, for *both* pleasure *and* bodily profit. I walk year around, just dressing differently for the differing seasons. My mind also wanders while walking. I actually "wrote" much of this book on such walks. Whether or not the book is good, I assure you that the walks were!

Another daily, yet year-round activity, that is substantially *less* active is *reading*. A writer is but a reader in reverse, and I am probably more of a reader than I am a writer. Like I have heard ballplayers say about *their* game, "I am also a fan."

If you have been enjoying reading this book, great! That's my aim. If you haven't—*my* fault—close it and go find a better one, because there are plenty of those. We could not in three lifetimes read all of the books worth reading. The world is filled with wonderful books, which makes it a wonderful place, at least sometimes, such as when we have the time and peace in which to read.

Since you are reading this, and likely prefer *not* to read about reading, I will not go on and on about it—you obviously already know all about it. It is now summer, so let's turn to some summer things worth doing—berry-picking, gardening, fishing. You will see at a glance that these are all, like walking and reading, *leisurely* pursuits—they strengthen the heart without straining it.

Bees have their stings and berry bushes have their thorns, making the honey and the berries all that much more precious. In my part of Ohio, black raspberries are ripe and ready from late June until a week or so after Independence Day, and the bigger blackberries ripen right after that, lasting through early August.

I spend hours harvesting both kinds of berries in a semi-wild area on the edge of town where my mother picked years before me, and where my grandfather picked them years before her. While my purple-stained fingers pluck my mind wanders, and more than a few stories have resulted from this activity—I *always* keep a memo-pad and pen handy while berrying. Should the pen run dry, I likely could use berry juice.

I could not go berrying last summer, because the chemo had so damaged my immune system that the unavoidable mosquito bites and thorn-scratches would have been not merely irritating but downright *dangerous*.

Those thorns are the berry plants' protection—the beautiful berries invite us to pluck and sample them, yet the thorny plants forbid us to trample them. This is security not against the intelligent humans but against the dumb and fingerless beasts that would trample the bushes, destroying the source of the berries that they devour.

That is a *reasonable* security system. Thinking of this while berrying recently, I thought of how *unreasonable* are so many of the security-minded ploys and plots of we humans—the reasoning creatures.

In the name of safety and security, many of our packaged goods need instructions on how to open them—what is called tamper-proof is often also opening-proof, not to mention nerve-wracking. Such packaging is supposedly aimed at preventing terrorist tampering with our junk food, but perhaps it *causes* terrorism by pissing off potential terrorists who cannot get at their Pop Tarts. Too many times trying to open something simple like peanut butter or a gizmo, I have muttered in frustration, *I paid for this and I want it open NOW!*

That is the relatively minor cost. In the name of security, we also allot huge chunks of our personal incomes to insurance against bad driving, bad people, and bad luck. For security against the intolerably terrible people, we even forfeit many of our collective freedoms. If only we could simply sprout thorns instead!

I went to some Little League baseball games this summer, and at two I found no bleachers upon which to sit. The second time, a local guy explained that the park or school that owned the field was told by their lawyers and insurers to get rid of the bleachers—someone *might* fall from them—and that this was happening at ball fields all around the country. When it is deemed so hazardous to watch them, I am amazed that they still allow the kids to play! Perhaps the youngsters would be "better off" (aka safer) staying home playing with their Gameboys or whatever while we oldsters safely sit nearby on the couch?

I think I better moderate some of my moderations. I self-imposed them "just to be safe," but safety is not the highest goal of humans, at least not this one. . .

If you have a garden, and a library, you have everything that you need. ~ Cicero

Berry season does not span the whole summer, but gardening season does. You ally up with God or with nature to grow a lovely and productive garden, but it is the *you* in that alliance who give shape to the growth.

Do not expect only growth and wholesomeness amongst the garden population, however. Some of the peppers will be hotheads, most of the cabbage hard-hearted, and all of the broccoli seedy. Many of the tomatoes become spoiled brats. As for the beans, you will find them too strung-out. No, do not expect wholesomeness in the garden. Even the veggies of higher character sometimes go bad.

Despite these character defects, or defective characters, the garden is a fine place to relax while getting some mild exercise doing productive activities. It is also a swell place to drink a beer or to read a book, or to drink many beers and read many books, albeit ideally not at the same time.

And, while I am dithering in my garden, reminding myself that zucchinis are technically *not* weeds to be yanked and chucked, I find a few earthworms, which I magically transform into *fish*-worms simply by dropping them into a dirt-filled cup.

Along with year-round reading and walking and summertime berrying and gardening, I also enjoy the three-season sport of fishing; all of these activities are good for the soul, meaning, methinks, the heart. Berrying I seek berries and gardening I seek veggies, but fishing I do not necessarily seek fish. No, I fish for a peaceful state of mind, and there is no catch-limit on that.

There *is,* however, a limit as to how much you can write about it without boring your reader, so let's go rather quickly to the best true-fishing story that I have netted …

I and my three cousins were young California men (I a transplanted Ohioan) and the things we did would have made us uninsurable if we cared to look into insurance, which we did not.

Safety and security be damned, one fine southern California day we inflated our two two-man rafts at Newport Beach; and we loaded those newly inflated rubber rafts with refreshments of a liquid nature and with fishing gear of a shark-fishing nature.

We struggled over the powerful breaker waves and then hitched a tow from a motorized dinghy out to the bobbing mile-marker buoy, to which we tied. Visible were sailboats further out to sea, and in the other direction, surfers riding the waves onto the now-distant beach; but we were all alone—except for what swam in the depths below us. We popped some tabs and started shark-fishing.

Oh, to be young and dumb, in love with living, and utterly uninsurable!

After an hour, my cousins in the other raft—Tim and Steve—caught a foot-long sand shark that would wind up, as we often did, pickled in alcohol, but in a high-school biology lab.

Another hour—and multiple popped tabs—later, my raft-partner Doug hooked into a substantially larger shark. He strained and strained until we could finally see a blue shark slightly longer than our raft struggling 20 feet below in the clear blue water.

As we started to urgently discuss cutting Doug's line, several sharks larger than the hooked one swam over to us. They presumably wished to see what the commotion was and whether it meant a bite to eat. I had just cautiously handed Doug the knife so that he could cut the line when the hooked shark saved him the effort by snapping that line.

Soon after that, safety and security being not entirely damned after all, we paddled rapidly toward shore and then gleefully raft-surfed the breaker-waves back onto the semi-solid sand of Newport Beach, where we impressed some sand-kneed Juniors with our junior sand shark.

And we walked across the beach-front boulevard into "The Crab-Cooker" fish-market/restaurant for some boiled shrimp requested by my Aunt Juli.

We gazed up at a station-wagon sized great white shark hanging from the ceiling, a shark with a tooth-lined mouth large enough to have nonchalantly swallowed us and our rafts in a single sharkly gulp.

We read *this* on a brass tag hanging from the shark's dirigible-sized belly:

CAUGHT 100 YARDS OFF OF THIS SAME BEACH

These days, summer days, when I am not berrying or gardening, you'll often find me wholeheartedly *cat*fishing from a mellow shore, perhaps reminiscing of a time when I lived a lifestyle on the edge of something more perilous, yet more promising—a time when I had not worried about insurance premiums, because I happily had nothing worth insuring in a premium life worth writing about, safety and security being secondary at best.

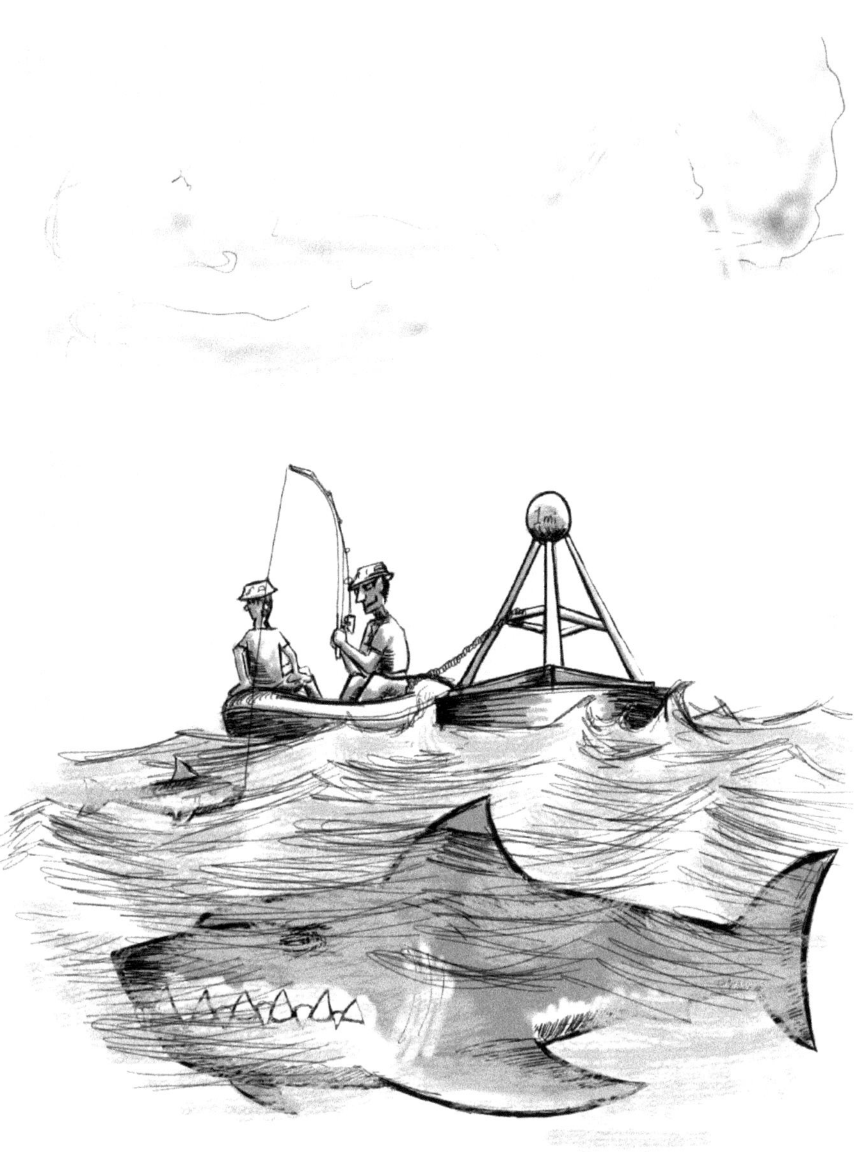

CHAPTER FOURTEEN

TIME IS A TRAIN, CHUGGING INTO MY STATION

Time is a stream I go a-fishing in.
~ Thoreau

Reliving that shark-fishing adventure was like a trip to my past—a past that now stretches back further than my foreseeable future stretches forward. Altogether, it is a microscopic drop in the stream of time. I do not think that Thoreau's philosophical metaphor above pertains to fishing for fish, and I picture him stationary as his stream of time flows past; it yet flows, and he yet stands there, thinking.

Time seems a fit topic for metaphor since its meaning is so hard to pin down in a tidy definition. Knowing that armchair philosophers lurk all about Facebook just waiting to pounce upon an opportunity to publicly philosophize, I sought amateur metaphors with this post: "Time is . . .?"

Here are some of my favorite posted responses:

- Time is a belt, looped around my bulging life.
- Time is a comedian with a killer punchline.
- Time is a stream running down my leg.
- Time is the bastard who stole my life.
- Time is a train, chugging into my station.

You can find philosophers eager to philosophize about time nearly anywhere and anytime. For instance, years ago in San Diego, I once conversed with a philosophical hobo. After lighting a smoke to mask his aroma and after complimenting him on his mild-weather choice of a city in which to establish his homelessness, I asked what had led him to his station in life.

I had expected to hear of childhood abuse or alcohol abuse, or a busted marriage or broken dreams; but I had instead heard this, dispensed in a surprisingly strong and steady voice: "Oh no, my friend—I *chose* this life; it did *not* choose me, nor did circumstances beyond my control corner me into it. I am a free man, a content one, fully employed in living life to the fullest."

"Oh," I had philosophized in return: "So *that* is your employment! It does not pay much, I suppose."

"Actually it pays me quite well in that which is priceless—my *time*," he had proudly replied.

"Well, have you ever tried trading some of that priceless commodity for some *cash*?" asked proudly employed I.

He had quizzically stared with surprisingly clear eyes and stroked his graying, crumb-laced beard awhile before replying, "Yes, I have at times, and I was ripped-off *every* time!"

"What? How? Sub-minimum wages?" I guessed, in an appropriately indignant tone.

"Any wages were a rip-off!" he had replied, as if I were an idiot, as perhaps I was. "Money is only good for buying *things*, and money and things are easily enough gotten and replaced. But my *time* is irreplaceable at *any* price. I could *not* buy it back with the money I received, or with any amount of money! It was *gone*—it and my self-respect!"

"So, now that you have your valued time back, what do you do with it," I had innocently asked, truly interested.

"Let me answer your naïve question with my own question: What primarily distinguishes humans from animals?"

"Um—oh, that's *easy*—the ability to take cow's milk and turn it into ice cream!"

"Besides that!" he had snapped, giving me a strange look. "I mean *the ability to think.* That is how I spend my valued time—and my thoughts are my own!"

I then handed him all of my pocket change, saying "Keep your time, sir, and use it to think all you want, but do get something to eat or drink." And *that* was my first philosophical life's lesson on the value of time. I had not known then its long-term effect on me, or I might have emptied my wallet for him, too. Instead, I had stood there watching him vanish into the stream of people passing by me.

Prisoners are also time-philosophers insofar as they refer to their court-imposed lifestyles as "doing time." What does that mean? It seems to add a wistful significance to it, like admitting that time is what has been taken from them or has been turned into something different than what it is on the "outside"—it has been turned into a punishment. In prison, one can only "kill" time—and I imagine the philosophical hobo muttering, "Murderers."

On the outside, where the use of time is more of an option than an imposition, one can "spend" it or "waste" it. Do not waste too much of it! To *spend* time, such as *spend some time with you*, hints at the value of time; so do the terms "make time" or "take time," the latter two maneuvers necessary when your time is otherwise already spent. *Spending time* is what the philosophical hobo does instead of spending the money for which he would *not* trade his time.

Free people—non-convicts—also will use the term, "killing time." When they use it around me, I want to ask them what they are a prisoner of that makes them want to kill time instead of spending time or making time. I do *not* say it, however, because I *myself* must sometimes do it, such as in medical office waiting rooms—plenty of *that* the past year; worse yet, for a few months last year "chemo brain" rendered me unable to read, a sure way to make spare time something to ""kill" rather than "spend." Since time will eventually kill us, purposefully "killing" it in the meanwhile only makes its inevitable victory more complete.

Maybe I am even more of a time philosopher than before, because I suddenly have less total time than what I had always expected, making it something even more valuable, making it something to spend wisely—which is why I am writing, hopefully not wasting my time and yours but instead making time stand still on these stationary pages.

I spend at least *some* of my treasured quiet time reading sci-fi tales of time-travel. Although science fiction *usually* has more fiction than it has science, the laws of nature, as interpreted by the laws of physics, do not rule out the possibility of time-travel. Current science actually holds out nearly as much hope for time-travel as it does for a chemo-less cancer-cure.

The Theory of Relativity's "time dilation" factor is central here—the closer that a person gets to the speed of light, the slower that time moves for that person. The reverse is likewise true. People at rest age more quickly—time passes more rapidly. Hence, a couch potato's beer or soda is *not* from the fountain of youth!

How do we take these scientific theories and actually build a time-machine? First, we have to get off of the couch! Second, we have to construct a "wormhole"—a tunnel connecting spatially separated sections of time-space. Third, we'll need to furnish the mouth of the wormhole with a sizeable velocity compared to the other end; and this will allow time-travel into the past simply by passing through the wormhole.

Easy, right? Now I am thinking of that hound dog Thoreau supposedly "fishing" in the stream of time. See the can of worms near his feet? Can you imagine the wormholes within it? David Henry Thoreau—a man ahead of his time *and* our time.

Using Thoreau's metaphor, along with the theories of modern physics and more than a little science fiction, I decided to build me a wormhole-enabled time machine. Beyond building the machine—no small challenge—my task was deciding to where, or to *when*, I would travel: past or future?

I try to not dwell in the past, but I would not mind *visiting* the past. What about a time-trip far back, easily bypassing all of recorded history, way back to the time of the primordial tide-pool that Aunt Rose had discussed? If I timed it right, I could arrive at the precise time when, according to scientists, life emerged from that heretofore inorganic pool. Yes, when Adam and Eve step out of it dripping, as if out of their own private Jacuzzi, I could await them. I would be prepared, offering towels that they might use to dry off, perhaps also to wrap around their wet naked bodies, at least Adam—I care *not* to see a naked dude, regardless of who he is or was! As for Eve, I would tell her the same thing that I tell my modern-day nieces: *don't talk to snakes*!

On the way back, I might stop in Elizabethan England and drop in on Shakespeare. I would like to chat with him, and maybe get the lowdown on the mysterious "Dark Lady"—the true identity of her (or him).

In addition, I contemplated a far-shorter trip to Dallas, Texas on a certain day in November of 1963, when and where I could lurk in the book depository or on the grassy knoll and detect what actually happened that historically dark day. Plus, while in 1963—20 years before the infamous Tylenol poisonings that led to "tamper-proof" (as in #%>*%# opening-proof) packaging—I would enjoy buying some Tylenol and, let's see, maybe some coffee creamer; and I would delight in simply opening them with ease, without broken fingernails or frayed nerves. Hopefully I could stop at that point. Hopefully, I would *not* compulsively-obsessively open package after package, a pile of opened, un-purchased packages piling up at my feet, as bewildered clerks call the 1963 cops.

I also considered traveling far into the future. By venturing into the misty distant future, say 100,000 years from now, I could discover what humankind had by then become, could see whether cancer had been conquered, poverty abolished, and war eradicated.

Then again, perhaps humans will not have even lasted that long? In that case, I would endeavor to learn what would happen, in a dehumanized world, to *cows*. I have sometimes wondered if cows could long-term survive *without* their hamburger-hungry keepers. It seems they might not be smart enough or fleet enough to endure outside of our fenced-in pastures. Plus, they are so damn *ugly*—I doubt that the speedy and splendid deer would care to interbreed with them. If the cows, nevertheless, would manage to flourish in a future world without humans to turn their milk into ice cream, then what higher purpose would they serve? I fear their lives would be meaningless in an ice cream-less world.

How about a much briefer trip to the near-future? I figured fifty years would suffice so that I could then scout around the local cemetery and hopefully locate my own tombstone. That way, I could unearth the yet-unknown date of my demise, and back to the present, plan accordingly. Then I thought perhaps that would be a bad idea. For one thing, I had never managed to, and did not expect to, pre-purchase a burial plot, meaning I will probably wind up, like Mozart, covered with lime in a paupers' grave. For another thing, it seems a lovely idea to keep living each day like it could be my last without actually knowing whether it will be or not. Plus, it may prove paradoxical, a living me visiting a dead me—what if I encounter a nephew or niece visiting (bless them!) the gravesite? That would definitely not do!

The near-future trip seemed like a bad idea.

In any case, just the other day I abandoned the entire time-travel project. I had discovered that my time-machine's worm-holes were all filled with worms. Interpreting that as a sign, I went fishing instead.

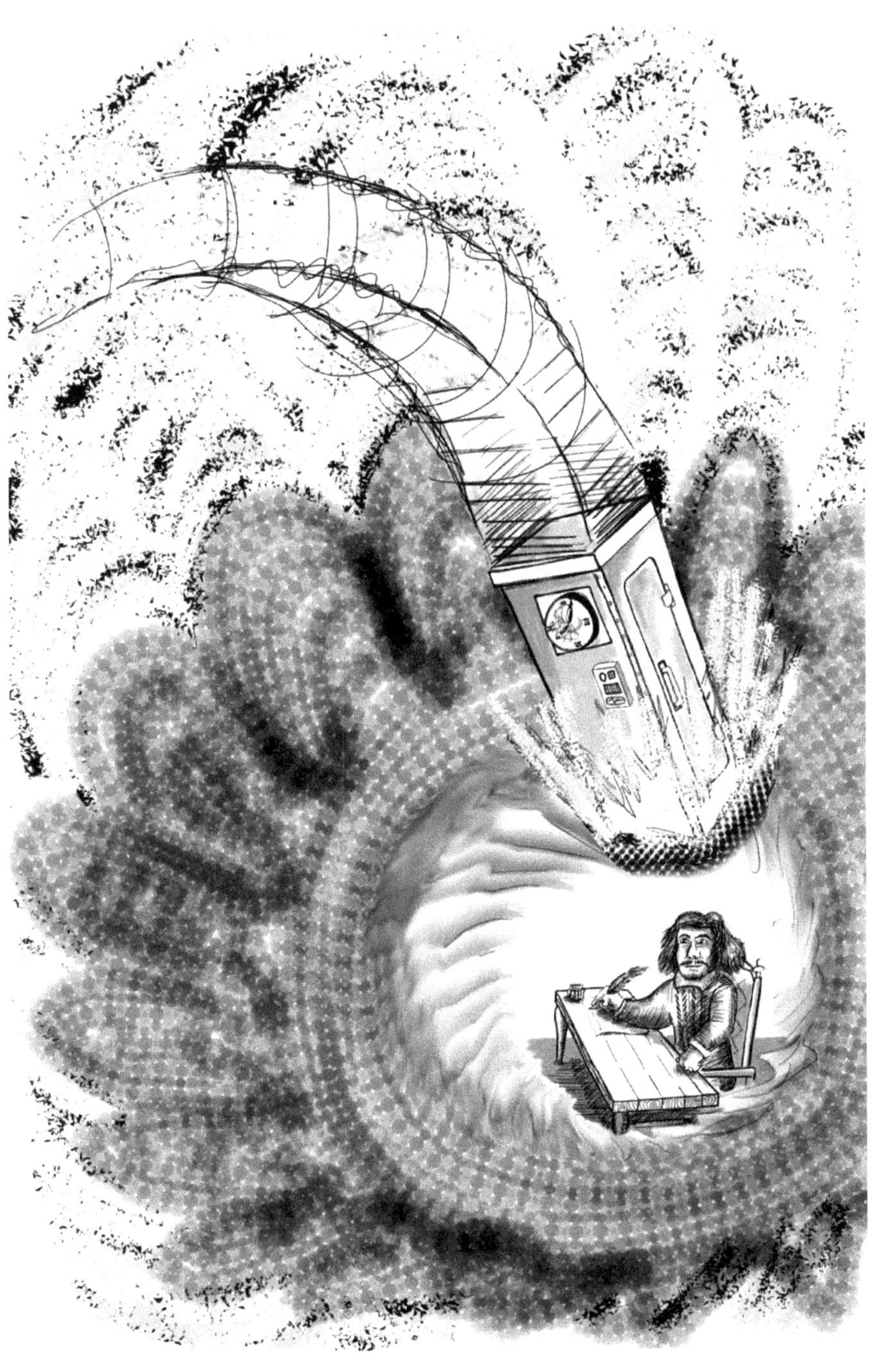

CHAPTER FIFTEEN

THE END

Life: A continuous series of disasters which result in one's death.
~ Anonymous

LATE-BREAKING NEWS-FLASH:

Last Tuesday, an echocardiogram revealed that the author's heart now pumps blood at near-normal levels.

Last Friday, a C-scan revealed that the author's cancer is mounting a comeback attempt.

Ah, here is my **F*** CANCER** tee-shirt—my **Still Ticking** tee will soon reside in my dust-rag bag. Done with what felt like a retreat, I am back to the battle—back to Facebook fame, back to special treatment, back to esteem-boosting warrior status. (As to the looming prospect of chemo and radiation, I will just have to put on my_big boy panties.) Plus, amidst all this excitement, a theme for my next book has emerged—*I'd Rather be Immortal.*

`I nonetheless need to prepare for The End—just in case—by putting my affairs in order. They have never been in order before, so that must be a good thing. Yes, it was time to see a liar, I mean lawyer. I searched the online yellow pages for local listings under *Attorneys—Wills, Trusts, Estate Planning.* After eliminating the lawyers I still owed for defending my youthful indiscretions, I reluctantly chose Attorney Richard "Dick" McMurphy who had attended (and often *not* attended) the same local high school as I had (and had not). I figured that even he could not screw up a simple will.

Way back then he had been the high school drunk. Times and people do change, though—now he is the town drunk. However, he does come from solid stock. His grandfather was a judge. His father is a judge. He is judged a shyster.

So it seemed appropriate when, at the top of the creaky wooden stairs on the second floor of a dilapidated old downtown office building, outside his office door, I saw this sign:

Good lawyers know the law

***Great* lawyers know the judge**

It was mausoleum-like quiet in the dusty building—it seemed like my prospective lawyer might be its only tenant. I cautiously prodded open the door, half-expecting to find a ghoulish scene behind it.

There sat Dick all alone, apparently plucking his eyelashes. I noticed all the signs of a seasoned drinker—a furrowed, puffy, flushed face; quivering hands and crumpled clothes; and, most telling of all, an open fifth of cheap bourbon on his surprisingly neat desktop—neat except for a pile of mutilated instant lotto tickets on its edge.

He unsteadily stood, smiled, and approached me while saying, "My man, it's been too long—how long?"

Without waiting for a reply, he opened his flabby arms as if for an embrace. No—a fake!—instead he reached up and delivered a noogie to the top of my head.

I said the same thing I had said countless times in the past, "Ow! That hurt, you creep!"

He chortled—bourbon vapors and cigar odors hovering head-high—and retreated back to his rickety chair, saying "Have a seat, *loser*."

Thinking *I'd rather have cancer than to be like you*, I sat on the safer-looking of the two low-slung chairs facing his steel desk, barely able to see beyond the front edge of it.

"I always used to see you walking around town," he said. "What happened?"

"Oh—I still walk a lot, but now not around town so much as on the park's walking paths. I recently got my driver's license," I said.

"Oh yea?" His eyes brightened behind their glaze overlay. "I also do DUIs, you know. . ."

I watched him chase that thought with a shot of bourbon.

"Actually, I don't drink much anymore, *Dick*. Maybe a glass or two of wine at home at the end of the day."

"Oh yea? Two glasses of what size?"

He eyed his own smudged and sizeable drinking jar, fingered an unlit half-cigar, and said, "So, you're here for *estate planning*? I heard about your cancer last year. It must've put the fright to ya, huh?"

He lit his cigar stub as well as the tips of a few stray strands of greasy grey hair, the reek of that really adding to the atmospheric stench.

I sat there trying to look immune to fright.

"Okay, okay," he finally said. "So, you've admitted that you're going to die someday. Well, welcome to the club."

He threw back another shot, flicked most of his lengthening ash into this silvery urn-looking thing on his desk, and added, "I should tell you that I am also an agent for Cherry-wood Cemetery here in town. As your counsel, I counsel you to consider pre-purchasing a burial plot there. Do it for your peace of mind—now *and* then."

"How do you know about that, Dick? Do you own a plot there?"

"Nope," he replied, nodding at the urn-like ashtray that he aimed at and missed, the ashes dropping instead into his nearly empty drinking jar. "I opt for cremation, and this here is my pre-purchased urn. I am prepping it for *my* ashes with cigar ashes—apropos, huh?"

He then extracted another smudged drinking jar from a lower drawer, saying, "You know why they bury lawyers twelve feet deep?"

I could think of a dozen reasons, but I bit at the bait: "Why?"

"Because deep down we really are good people!" He chortled.

I grinned, and he pushed some papers my way.

"Sign these, write me a check for, let's see, a cool grand, and I'll make you the proud owner of a fine plot, possibly beneath a cherry tree. If I'm right, you've never owned property—here's your chance!"

"I don't know Dick, I've spent half my life trying to disassociate myself from this town, so why would I want to spend *forever* here?"

"Um—cuz it's a great place to raise kids?"

"Raise *crack-heads*, you must mean."

"Look here, my man, property values are rising again—look at it as an investment in your future!"

"Yea, rents are rising, too," I mused.

Suddenly an image wandered into mind, a peaceful image of my pup tent pitched on my new property, surrounded by the headstones of permanently sleeping neighbors.

"Okay, I'll do it," I said, grabbing a pen, then another, and yet another, until I finally found one, a red one that worked.

After we finished the paperwork on that, resulting in my having a deed to my first and last piece of property, he said, "I guess you also want to write a will? Did you bring those documents that I requested?"

"Sure did," I responded, pushing some of them his way. "Those show my current royalty earnings as well as my savings and investments for the past ten years. I've also listed my, um, assets."

As he read, sipped, puffed, and flicked errant ashes, a smile appeared on his flaccid face; and it grew and grew until, finally, he chortled, choked, recovered and said, "Man, I figured with all those books you have out there, what is it, six, seven, hell, I figured you had it *made*. Instead, I find you're just another starving artist, or would be starving except you're clearly eligible for food stamps!"

He wiped his brow with a filthy hanky, downed another shot, refilled the jar and slid it my way.

After wiping its rim with my shirt, I drank—it tasted ashy.

"Well," I said, "Maybe book sales will pick up after I'm gone! You know, I've always thought of my *books* as being my headstones. As such, I have my headstones on bookshelves all over the world. The world is my graveyard!"

That gave him another chuckle, and I chuckled too. His own metaphorical headstone would be what? A court order or a divorce decree, an eviction notice or stock certificate?

He set to work, adding, subtracting, and filling in the blanks on the will, which was also rather ashy by now. Finally, he gathered all of the papers, stacked them neatly—and then crumpled them into a big ball, which he tossed toward the nearby trashcan.

What? "What'd you do that?"

Leering at me, he replied, "After deducting all of my fees for today's consultation, you have no assets—they're all *mine*!"

"Okay, *Dick*."

Rising, I eyed the drunken shyster. I knew that *he* knew that he would still have to account in the will for future royalties of unknown amounts: 15 cents, fifteen bucks, fifteen thousand (ha ha), who knows? Who cares?

"Just mail me the final version." I then walked out and into a splendid eve, walked while trying to recall where I had stored that pup tent.

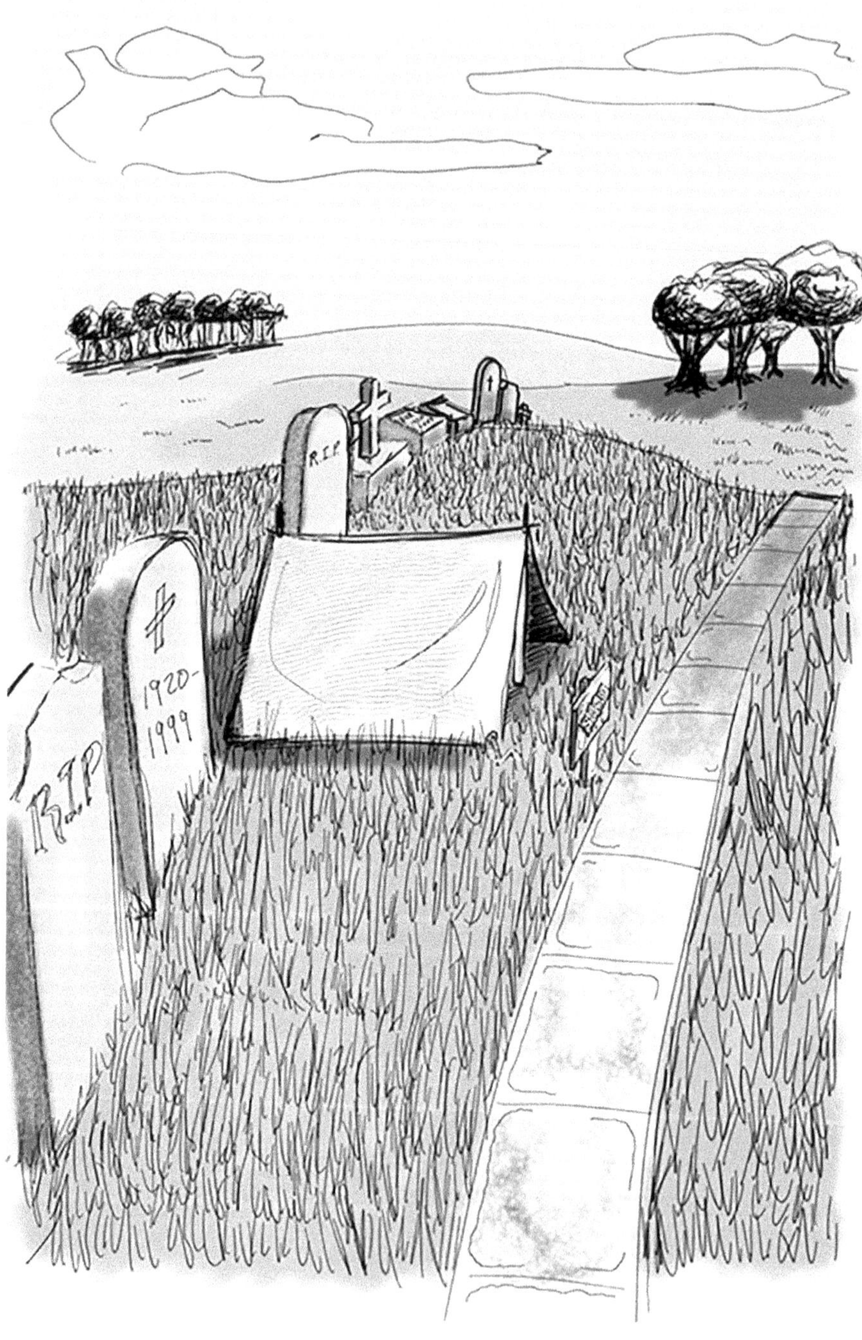
R.I.P.
1920-
1999
R.I.P

www.ingramcontent.com/pod-product-compliance
Ingram Content Group UK Ltd.
Pitfield, Milton Keynes, MK11 3LW, UK
UKHW020151200726
13856UKWH00003B/941

9 781614 772484